COOKBOOK
for Weaners

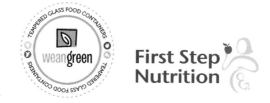

Forward To Cookbook

Congratulations on your new baby- can you believe it's time to start solids already?! Of course you want the best for your baby. One of the most important jobs you have as a parent is feeding your baby! What (and how) you feed your baby, effects not only their current energy level and nutrient status. It also effects their tendency to be a picky eater, their lifelong physical health and lifelong emotional relationship with food.

As the mother of two young children and a Registered Dietitian, I know the importance of making your own baby food. While you can find some healthy pre-made baby foods, there are always benefits to making your own, including:

- Teaching children that homemade foods are enjoyable and the easiest choice.

- Saving money.

- Allowing your baby to eat a greater variety of food.

- Progressing the texture in your baby's food.

- Using breast milk, instead of water to make your baby food.

Starting solids is a fun and exciting time for both you and your baby. Here are some tips to make the process go smoothly:

- Listen to your baby regarding the amount they want to eat. More? Ok! Nothing? Ok too!

- Iron is the most important nutrient for your baby at this stage. Meat contains iron in its most easily absorbable form, and even makes a great first food! Try to have an iron source at most meals (meat, fish, beans, eggs or fortified cereal).

- Let your baby feed themselves and be messy. This is part of the learning process!

- Progress with increasing the texture of your baby food, and adding finger foods.

Following Wean Green's tips and recipes in this book will make it easy for you to prepare delicious and nutritious meals for your little one. Good luck, and have fun!!

Jennifer House MSc, RD & mom of 2

www.firststepnutrition.com

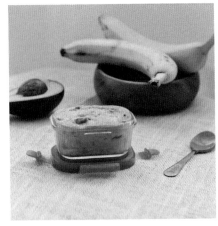 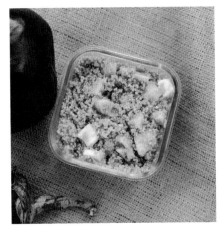 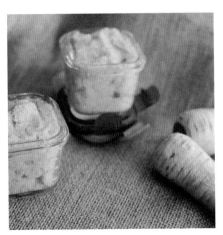

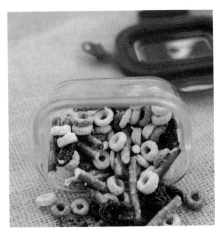 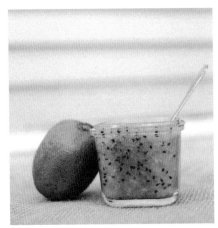 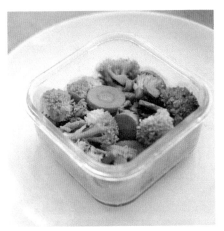

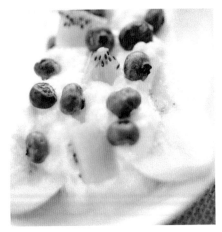 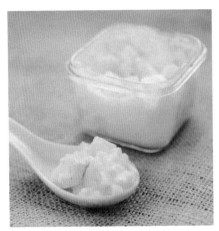 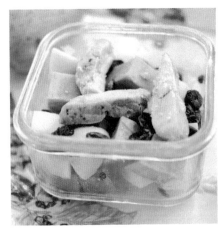

Introduction

Melissa Gunning & The Wean Green Team

As you have been enjoying the first six months of parenthood your little weaner has been watching you enjoy all sorts of foods. Now your weaner is getting curious and is eager to start eating all those delicious smelling foods too. Lucky you! You are in complete control of what goes into that little weaner's body and our job is to help you do it right!

The reason we wrote this book is that we were in the same position as you not that long ago and had no clue where to start. We found many great resources but they seemed to be so scattered and to require so much effort every time we were looking for a new recipe. We hope that you get what you require out of this book, we had a blast creating it and our little testers have helped us test all the recipes ourselves. Yep, that's right, we ate a lot of baby food to get you this book.

Why make your own baby food? There are so many answers to that question. Mainly we say it is to show off your super mama skills in the kitchen and fill that baby with the healthiest foods your gardens and markets have to offer. And it's cheaper! With this said, we know you're busy and we are here to help you make this a fun and fulfilling (literally) task.

Are you ready to create a weaner? Remember, all babies are not created equally, and you should check with your health care provider before introducing solid foods!

My Mother's Grandma's Great Grandma Told Her...

Well, considering our mothers' mothers believed that a little bit of whisky went a long way in soothing a new baby, we are not going to use all of the advice we received when our weaners arrived. We believe that the old "rules" for feeding babies are just guidelines now. Many of the rules have changed, and mom's intuition and weaner's cues should be a contributing factor in introducing solids. Following are some good guidelines to consider.

Is Your Baby Ready to Join the Weaner Club? There Is No Rush!

Babies should be breastfed and/or formula fed exclusively for the first 6 months of their lives. The World Health Organization (WHO) suggests that once babies reach the age of 6 months, they are ready to become weaners. There are disadvantages to starting solids too early (for instance, your baby won't get the full immunity and allergy protection from breast milk) or too late (your baby needs extra iron and nutrients at around 6 months). We won't argue with the WHO, but really the final decision is in your hands, and your weaner's desire to join the not-so-elite club of eating solids.

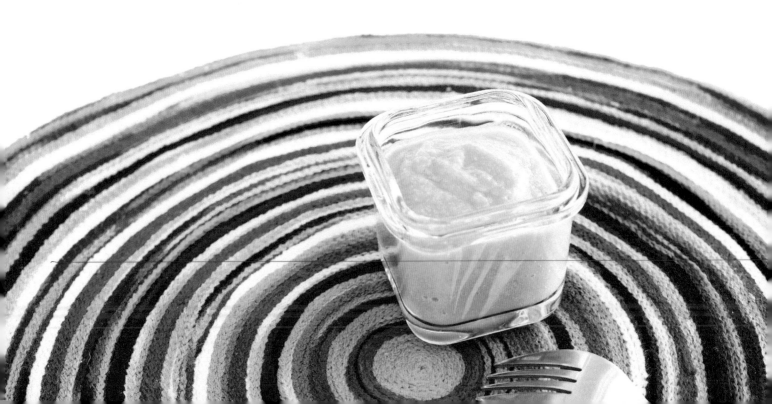

Being a parent automatically qualifies you to be a master mind and body language reader! These are the telltale signs that your baby is ready for those first foods:

- When they are able to sit up in the highchair without support and hold up their disproportionately sized head

- When they are able to show signs that they are no longer hungry, including turning away from the spoon or, one of our personal favorites, throwing it on the floor

- When they can swallow food instead of reflexively pushing it out with their tongue

- When that longing look is no longer solely aimed on their beautiful mama's eyes and more focused on what their beautiful mamas are putting into their mouths. Some babies even grab out for the food that they see people eating.

Be Aware of Allergies

Babies are sensitive little people. Even though everyone seems to know someone whose baby has a food allergy it is reported that only about 4% to 8% of children have a true food allergy! The Big Eight most allergenic foods are cow's milk, eggs, tree nuts, peanuts, wheat, fish, shellfish, and soy. While official recommendations no longer cite any evidence that delaying these foods will prevent allergy, you should still watch your baby carefully after introducing these foods.

If your weaner develops hives, swelling, red patches, tummy pains, vomiting, or diarrhea, call your health care provider immediately. More severe reactions can result in anaphylaxis, which includes wheezing, swelling of the tongue and mouth, and trouble breathing. If your weaner develops any of these symptoms, seek emergency medical assistance immediately.

The "Wait Three Days" Rule

Food needs to be introduced to our little weaners gradually. You should always wait at least three days in between introducing new foods. It is how you monitor baby's reactions to solids, and will help you determine which food they are allergic to if they have a reaction.

Outlaws

Honey is outlawed for your weaner until after their first birthday. It can cause botulism (food poisoning) which can be fatal in infants.

It is still a routine recommendation to avoid dairy products until at least 9 months of age. You will have plenty of other foods to introduce to your weaner before that so we have waited for the 9–12 month section to introduce cow's milk products. We have also waited to introduce egg white until 9 months. Egg yolks and whites contain different proteins,so they should be introduced separately.

Other than that, if there is no family risk of food allergy you do not need to outlaw any foods once your baby starts solids. If your weaner does show signs of food allergy, or has a parent or sibling with food allergies, your health care professional may have a different recommendation.

Use Organic Foods

Organic foods are categorized as foods that are free of insect-killing pesticides, unnatural fertilizers, hormones, antibiotics, or biotechnology products. Many people question the benefit of buying organic. As a bonus, organic produce has higher antioxidant levels, which, according to scientific research, could help fight cancer. Organic farming practices are also far more environmentally responsible—and we want to preserve our beautiful earth for our children's sake!

Sometimes organic foods are not available for certain foods at certain times. Try and stock up if you see something that is not normally at your market or grocer—or if you are even keener, your garden!

If you choose to purchase conventional foods instead of organic, beware of the so-called "dirty dozen." The Environmental Working Group's Shopper's Guide to Pesticides lists the following 12 fruits and vegetables as having the highest pesticide residues »

Dirty Dozen Plus™ Buy these organic

1 Apples

2 Celery

3 Sweet bell peppers

4 Peaches

5 Strawberries

6 Nectarines - imported

7 Grapes

8 Spinach

9 Lettuce

10 Cucumbers

11 Blueberries - domestic

12 Potatoes

Plus

+ Green beans

+ Kale/Greens

+ May contain pesticide residues of special concern

Equipment Needed to Make Baby Food

- Cutting board
- Vegetable peeler
- Large knife
- Paring knife
- Small saucepan
- Large saucepan
- Wooden spoon
- Measuring cups and spoons
- Wean Cubes

- Marker to label your Wean Cubes
- Food processor, Magic Bullet, or blender
- Steamer basket
- Potato masher
- Loaf pan
- Baking dish
- Slow cooker
- Whisk
- Colander

Preparing, Storing, and Serving Your Homemade Creations

Set aside some time to make a few different foods at once. It is so nice to spend an hour in the kitchen and have a week's worth of food for your weaner.

NOTE:

Don't make too-too much of one puree, as your weaner will be eating pureed food for only a short while, before you will add in some lumps and more texture. If you do have leftover purees, you can add them to big-kid food. Try mixing one of the purees into your next veggie sauce, soup, or stew. And use leftover pureed fruits in a smoothie or mixed with plain yogurt!

PREPARING:

Make sure you wash all fruits and veggies well, as well as your hands and cooking tools. Trim the fat off of meat and peel fruits and veggies according to the recipe.

STORING:

Wean Cubes were designed for this purpose. After your big batch of food is cooked, let it cool and then pour it into the Wean Cubes. Portion sizes are up to your weaner. Start with about 1/2 to 1 ounce and continue up from there. Don't forget to leave some room for expansion if you are freezing.

If you will not be using your Wean Cubes within 2 to 3 days, they should go in the freezer; otherwise the fridge is fine. Use a marker (it will wipe right off after, even if it's permanent) to write the date and contents on the front of the Wean Cube. Generally you should not leave purees in the freezer longer than 3 months.

SERVING:

Wean Cubes were invented with serving as a primary use. They are made of tempered glass that does not leach chemicals into the food. If you are serving a newly cooked masterpiece puree, make sure you allow it to cool to room temp. We recommend thawing foods in the refrigerator overnight, so they are ready for a quick reheat in the morning. If you don't have time, you can throw them directly into the microwave from the freezer. It normally takes 15 to 30 seconds to reheat your weaner's food to the right temperature from the fridge, and 30 to 60 seconds when you are thawing it from the freezer. Make sure you stir it well, and ensure that it is not too hot. Once you have defrosted your food, don't refreeze it.

NOTE:

Glass is not designed to withstand extreme temperature changes. Do not put your frozen Wean Cube in hot water to warm it, as the glass may break.

6-9 Months

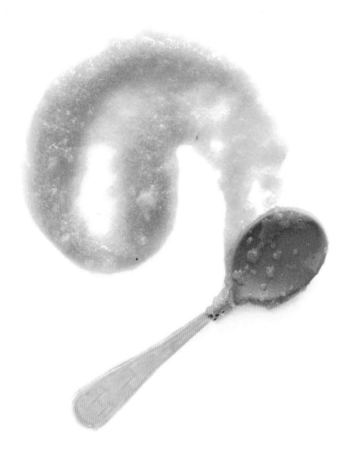

This is where it all begins. . . . Every Good Food Deserves a Nice Drink Pairing

Starting solids does not mean that you are replacing baby's breast milk or formula (yet). It is important that you do not reduce your weaner's daily milk intake, as it is very important for growth and development. At this stage you are simply introducing a foreign concept, to let your baby experiment. Water is not necessary at this time but you can introduce a few sips to baby in a cup. Make sure that water is not replacing breast milk.

How Much Should Your Weaner Eat?

The only person who can answer this question accurately is your weaner! For the first couple of meals it may be only a teaspoon or they may refuse solids all together. Start with a serving of 1 ounce and continue from there. Weaners will tell you when they are done. One day they may eat 3 ounces and the next they may barely finish 1/2 ounce. Don't worry—it's normal!

Start with one meal a day and work your way up from there. Breakfast is the best time to start solids. That way you will have the rest of the day to watch your baby for signs of food allergy and they are likely to be most hungry in the morning. Around 7–8 months, you can add a second meal, and at 8–9 months, three meals per day. By the time your little weaner turns one year old they will be eating a similar pattern to you: three meals and a few snacks per day.

WEANER'S AGE	APPROXIMATE CALORIE NEEDS FROM FOOD	NUMBER OF TIMES TO OFFER SOLIDS PER DAY
6–8 months	200 calories	6 months: 1 meal 7 months: 2 meals 8 months: 2–3 meals Continue to offer breast milk or formula on demand.
9–11 months	300 calories	3 meals (snacks optional) Continue to offer breast milk or formula on demand.
12–14 months	550 calories	3 meals and 2–3 snacks

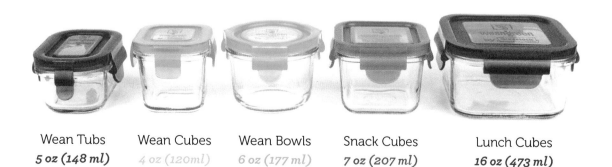

Wean Tubs	Wean Cubes	Wean Bowls	Snack Cubes	Lunch Cubes
5 oz (148 ml)	*4 oz (120ml)*	*6 oz (177 ml)*	*7 oz (207 ml)*	*16 oz (473 ml)*

Sugar and Spice: Not Necessarily Nice

Bland food? Don't worry about it! Your weaner does not need any added sugar or salt. Foods high in sugar and salt are often low in nutrients. Your weaner's kidneys are not mature enough to handle an excess of salt. As for spice, it is okay to offer your baby "plain" foods first, so that they can get accustomed to some gentle flavors. Then, if they accept and enjoy some spices, it is not harmful to add salt-free spices such as cinnamon, nutmeg, or oregano. In fact, adding some of these "adult" herbs and spices may expand your weaner's palate, and make them less likely to be picky later on.

Picky Eaters?

Nope. Not picky, just not interested. This is all brand new to your weaner. Just because your weaner doesn't want something one day does not mean that they will not try it the next day! Continue to offer your baby a rounded diet.

One of our weaners wouldn't eat avocado until she was well past 10 months, and now it is one of her favorite foods! As the parent, you decide what food your weaner eats (don't bring out their favorite food as back-up!). And they decide how much of that food they want to eat.

Meat Is a Great First Food —Really!

It's important that your weaner's first foods contain iron. Your 7- to 12-month-old needs 11 mg of iron daily—more than an adult male! Iron is important for brain development, so they can learn and have energy. And at around 6 months of age, your little weaner's stores of iron from before birth are running out. Good sources of iron are iron-fortified infant cereals, meats, legumes, and egg yolks. The type of iron in meat is absorbed better than the iron in fortified cereals and other foods. So meat is a great first food choice for baby! It is not hard for your weaner to digest meat, and they are unlikely to be allergic to it. How many people do you know who have a meat allergy? Probably none, but it is possible you know someone with a grain allergy such as celiac disease. Another great reason to start with meat!

Progress That Puree!

First foods should be very smooth in texture. You create this by blending thoroughly and adding more liquid. Once your baby has adapted to this texture, you can start to make the food chunkier. Add less liquid and/or blend less. It's easy to do when you are making your own food!

Choking Prevention

As your weaner progresses throughout this book you will serve chunkier foods. It is common for babies to gag on new textures. Stay calm, and just know that gagging is not the same as choking. It is a part of learning how to eat, and brings the food back up for your baby to chew it more! If you overreact, you might scare your weaner. However, choking is a real risk as your baby will not be able to breathe and will not be making any noise. Take an infant CPR class and avoid choking hazards.

Foods that are considered choking hazards: whole nuts, seeds, fish with bones, grapes, hard veggies, chewy meats, raisins, dried fruit, candy, pomegranates, hot dogs, sausage, frozen bananas, popcorn, cheese slices, celery, and long pasta like spaghetti.

As a rule of thumb, do not serve foods that are round: grapes, cherry tomatoes, and other soft fruits and veggie balls should be cut into quarters. Hard fruits and veggies should be diced, shredded, or pureed.

The "Wait Three Days" Rule

Remember to wait three days between introducing new foods so you can link any allergic reaction to a specific food.

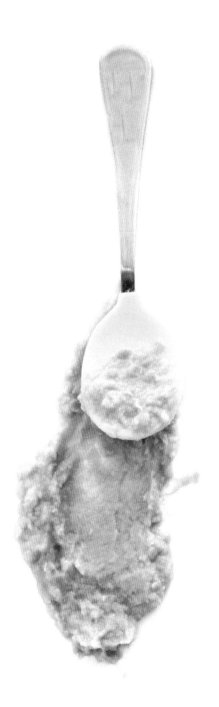

Sample Meal Plan: 6 Months

The following sample meal plan will help introduce new foods to your weaner for the first month of solids. This takes into account introducing a new food every three days. Once you have tried a food, you can continue with that food, while you add a new food. For example, on days 4–6, you can offer Bison Puree and Sweet Potato Puree. Continue to provide breastmilk and/or formula on demand.

All recipes can be found in the 6-9 month section of this book.

	BREAKFAST (new foods bold)
Days 1–3	**Bison Puree**
Days 4–6	**Sweet Potato Puree** + Bison Puree
Days 7–9	**Kidney Bean Puree** + Sweet Potato Puree
Days 10–12	**Roasted Apple Puree** + Bison Puree
Days 13–15	**Pear Mush** + Kidney Bean Puree
Days 16–18	**Green Bean Puree** + Bison Puree
Days 19–21	**Roasted Nectarine Puree** + Kidney Bean Puree
Days 22–24	**Kamut Cereal** + Pear Mush
Days 25–27	**Plum Puree** + Bison Puree

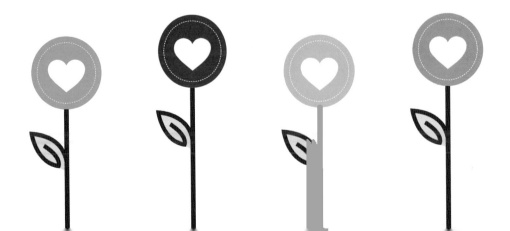

Sample Meal Plan: 7–8 Months

This sample meal plan takes you through months 7 and 8. You will continue to offer a new food for breakfast every three days as well as adding a second meal. Notice that at least one iron source has been offered per day (meat, legumes, or egg yolk), as this is the most important nutrient for your weaner to get from solid foods at this stage. Continue to provide breastmilk and/or formula on demand.

All recipes can be found in the 6-9 month section of this book.

	BREAKFAST (new foods bold)	LUNCH OR DINNER ("OLD" foods)
Month 7 Days 1–3	**Chicken Puree** + Roasted Apple Puree	Pear Mush + Kidney Bean Puree
Days 4–6	**Avocado Mush** + Kamut Cereal	Bison Puree + Green Bean Puree
Days 7–9	Slow Cooker Baby Breakfast (made with **brown rice**)	Chicken Puree + Broccoli Puree
Days 10–12	**Lentil Puree** + Plum Puree	Bison Puree + Sweet Potato Puree
Days 13–15	**Butternut Squash Puree** + Chicken Puree	Lentil Puree + Avocado Mush
Days 16–18	**Egg Yolk** + Pear Mush	Chicken Puree + Plum Puree
Days 19–21	**Acorn Squash Puree** and Roasted Nectarine Puree	Egg Yolk + Butternut Squash Puree
Days 22–24	**Pork Tenderloin Puree** + Sweet Potato Puree	Brown Rice Cereal + Roasted Nectarine Puree
Days 25–27	**Roasted Peach Puree** + Brown Rice Cereal	Lentil Puree + Pear Mush
Days 28–30	**Cantaloupe Mush** + Kamut Cereal	Pork Tenderloin Puree + Green Bean Puree
Month 8 Days 1–3	**Tofu Mush** + Green Bean Puree	Sweet Chicken
Days 4–6	**Mango Puree** + Chicken Puree	Tofu Mush + Cantaloupe Mush
Days 7–9	**Chickpea Puree** + Butternut Squash Puree	Smashed Baby Burgers + Mango Puree
Days 10–12	**Spinach Puree** + Pork Tenderloin Puree	Chickpea Puree + Avocado Mush
Days 13–15	Tofu **Banana** Wheat Germ*	Lentil Puree + Spinach Puree
Days 16–18	**Quinoa Cereal** + Roasted Peach Puree	Egg Yolk + Plum Puree
Days 19–21	Slow Cooker **Apricot** Chicken Meal	Pork Tenderloin Puree + Butternut Squash Puree
Days 22–24	**Carrot Puree** + Egg Yolk	Quinoa Cereal + Pear Mush
Days 25–27	**Top Sirloin Roast Puree** + Cantaloupe Mush	Baked Chicken and Carrots
Days 28–30	**Pumpkin** and Carrot Mush + Chickpea Puree	Tofu Mush + Mango Puree

*Your baby has had wheat, since Kamut is a type of wheat.

There is a lot of food here, and you may not introduce it all before you get to the next stage. That is okay; you have many years to introduce your weaner to all of the wonderful foods out there!

CEREALS

Cereal Powder

Do not serve these powders uncooked; they are for use in the recipes that follow. You can use brown rice, old-fashioned rolled oats (not quick-cooking oats), barley, Kamut, or quinoa, but do not mix different types of grains in the same batch.

1. Place the uncooked dry grain in your blender and blend until there are no chunks left. It should be a fine powder.

2. Store the powder in a cool, dry area for up to 2 months in a tightly sealed Wean Cube.

Barley Cereal

1¼ cups water

½ cup homemade
barley powder

(see Cereal Powder recipe on page 19)

1. Bring the water to a boil in a 2-quart saucepan over high heat.

2. Using your whisk, stir in the barley powder.

3. Turn the heat down to medium.

4. Whisk constantly for 10 minutes.

5. There is no need to puree; the whisking will produce the correct consistency for your weaner.

Kamut Cereal

1¼ cups water

½ cup homemade
Kamut powder

(see Cereal Powder recipe on page 19)

1. Bring the water to a boil in a 2-quart saucepan over high heat.

2. Using your whisk, stir in the Kamut powder.

3. Turn the heat down to medium.

4. Whisk constantly for 10 minutes.

5. There is no need to puree; the whisking will produce the correct consistency for your weaner.

Brown Rice Cereal

1¼ cups water

½ cup homemade
brown rice powder

(see Cereal Powder recipe on page 19)

1. Bring the water to a boil in a 2-quart saucepan over high heat.

2. Using your whisk, stir in the rice powder.

3. Turn the heat down to medium.

4. Whisk constantly for 10 minutes.

5. There is no need to puree; the whisking will produce the correct consistency for your weaner.

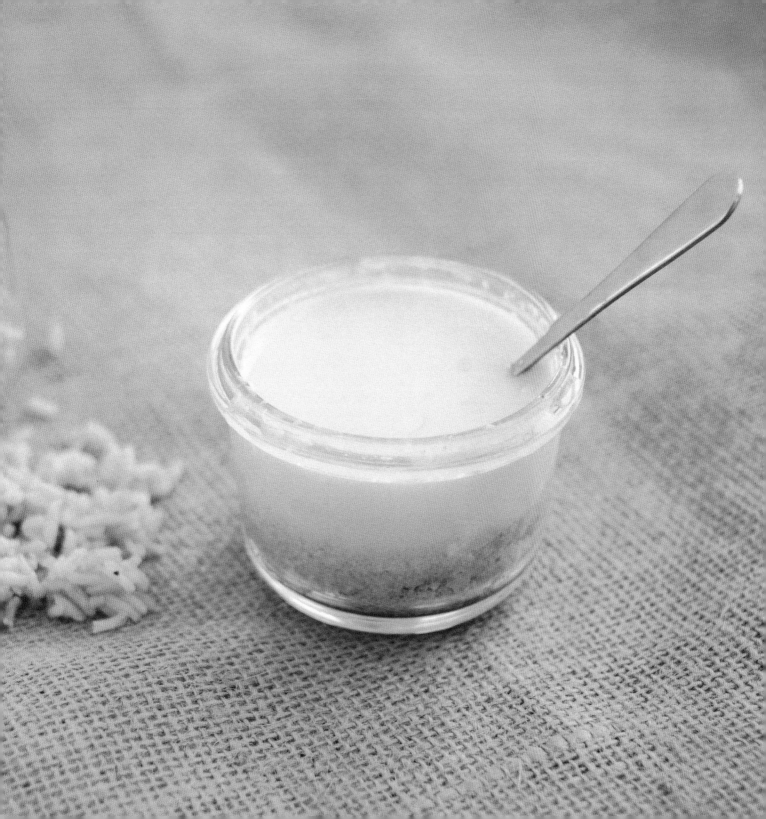

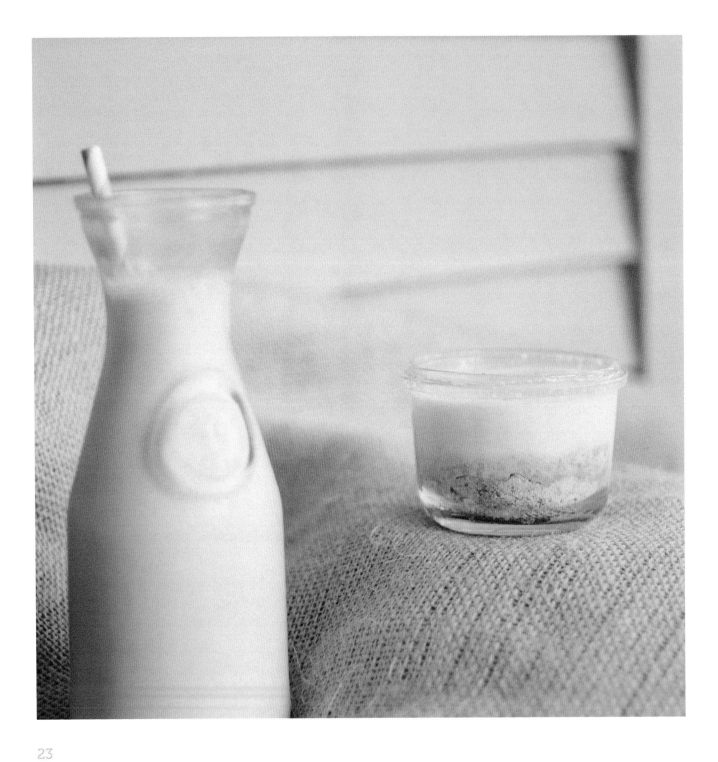

Oatmeal Cereal

1¼ *cups water*

½ *cup homemade*
   oatmeal powder

   (see Cereal Powder recipe on page 19)

1. Bring the water to a boil in a 2-quart saucepan over high heat.

2. Using your whisk, stir in the oatmeal powder.

3. Turn the heat down to medium.

4. Whisk constantly for 10 minutes.

5. There is no need to puree; the whisking will produce the correct consistency for your weaner.

Quinoa Cereal

1¼ cups water

**½ cup homemade
quinoa powder**
(see Cereal Powder recipe on page 19)

1. Bring the water to a boil in a 2-quart saucepan.

2. Using your whisk, stir in the quinoa powder.

3. Turn the heat down to medium.

4. Whisk constantly for 10 minutes.

5. There is no need to puree; the whisking will produce the correct consistency for your weaner.

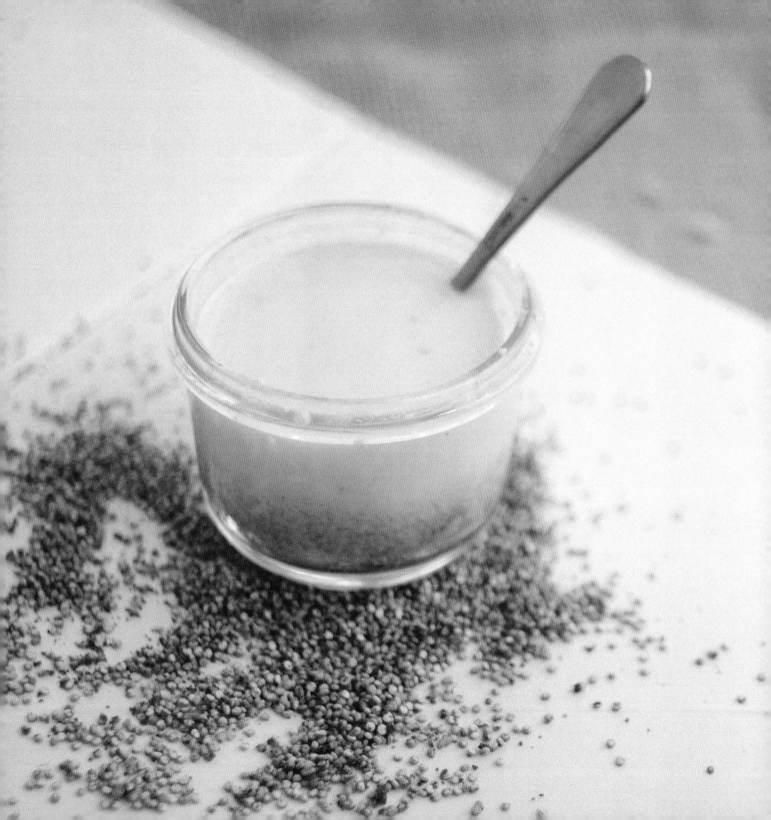

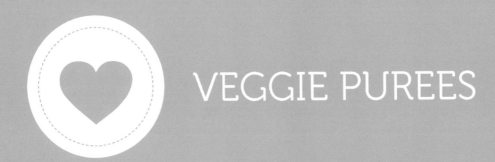

VEGGIE PUREES

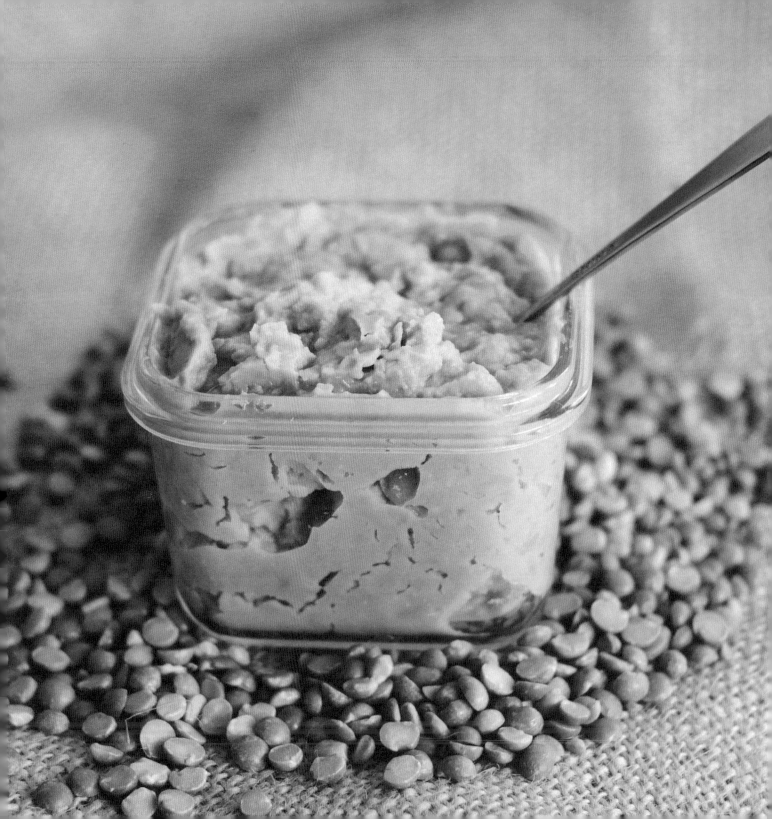

Pea Puree

*2 cups peas,
fresh or frozen*

1. Place a steamer basket in a pot and add enough water to just touch the bottom of the steamer basket.

2. Cover the pot and bring the water to a boil over high heat.

3. Add the peas, turn the heat down to medium, and loosely cover the pot.

4. Steam for 3 to 5 minutes, until the peas are very soft. Allow to cool slightly.

5. Puree in a food processor or blender, adding breast milk or cooking water as needed to achieve the desired consistency.

Sweet Potato Puree

4 sweet potatoes

1. Preheat the oven to 400°F.

2. Poke the sweet potatoes with a fork, seven times each.

3. Wrap each sweet potato in foil and place directly on the middle oven rack. Bake for 1 hour.

4. Allow to cool slightly. Unwrap the sweet potatoes, cut them in half, and then pull off the skins.

5. Puree in a food processor or blender, adding breast milk or water as needed to achieve the desired consistency.

Green Bean Puree

1 pound green beans, ends trimmed

1. Place a steamer basket in a pot and add enough water to just touch the bottom of the steamer basket.

2. Cover the pot and bring the water to a boil over high heat.

3. Add the green beans, turn down the heat to medium, and loosely cover the pot.

4. Steam for about 15 minutes, or until the beans are very soft. Allow to cool slightly.

5. Puree in a food processor or blender, adding breast milk or cooking water as needed to achieve the desired consistency.

Butternut Squash Puree

1 butternut squash,
cut in half lengthwise
and seeded

1. Preheat the oven to 400°F.

2. Put the squash in a baking pan, cut sides down, with just enough water to cover the bottom.

3. Bake for 45 minutes.

4. Allow to cool slightly. Scoop out the squash from the skin.

5. Puree in a food processor or blender, adding breast milk or water as needed to achieve the desired consistency.

Acorn Squash Puree

1 acorn squash,
cut in half and seeded

1. Preheat the oven to 400°F.

2. Put the squash in a baking pan, cut sides down, with just enough water to cover the bottom.

3. Bake for 45 minutes.

4. Allow to cool slightly. Scoop out the squash from the skin.

5. Puree in a food processor or blender, adding breast milk or water as needed to achieve the desired consistency.

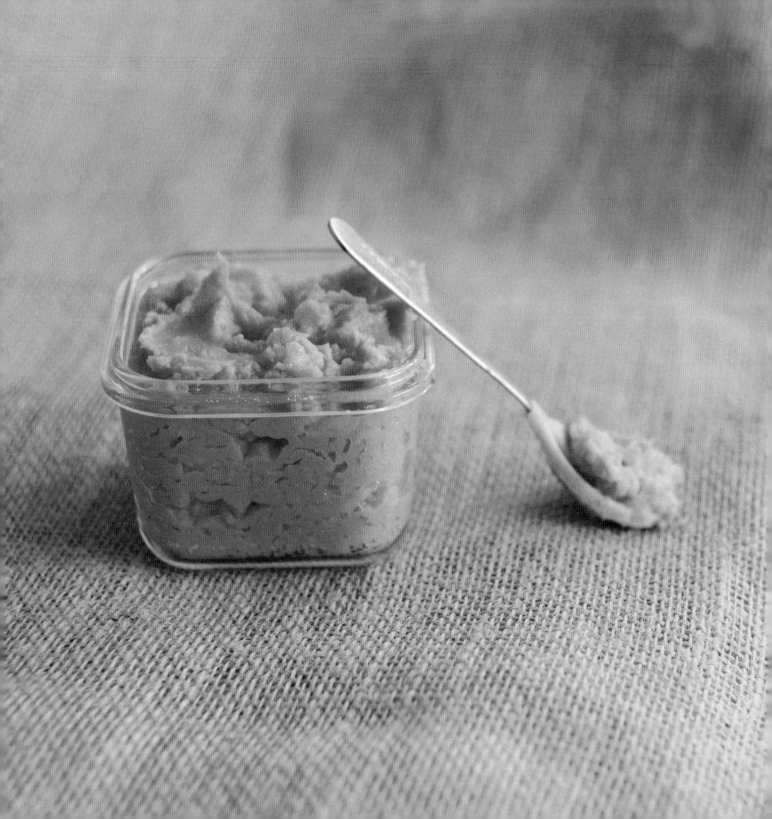

Pumpkin Puree

*1 pumpkin,
cut in half and gutted*

1. Preheat the oven to 400°F.

2. Put the pumpkin in a baking pan, cut sides down, with just enough water to cover the bottom.

3. Bake for 45 minutes.

4. Allow to cool slightly. Scoop out the pumpkin from the skin.

5. Puree in a food processor or blender, adding breast milk or water as needed to achieve the desired consistency.

Carrot Puree

*10 carrots, peeled and
cut into chunks*

1. Place a steamer basket in a pot and add enough water to just touch the bottom of the steamer basket.

2. Cover the pot and bring the water to a boil over high heat.

3. Add the carrots, turn the heat down to medium, and loosely cover the pot.

4. Steam for 6 to 8 minutes, or until the carrots are very soft. Allow to cool slightly.

5. Puree in a food processor or blender, adding breast milk or cooking water as needed to achieve the desired consistency.

Yellow Squash Puree

*1 yellow squash, peeled
and cut into large pieces*

1. Place a steamer basket in a pot and add enough water to just touch the bottom of the steamer basket.

2. Cover the pot and bring the water to a boil over high heat.

3. Add the squash, turn the heat down to medium, and loosely cover the pot.

4. Steam for 3 to 5 minutes, or until the squash is very soft. Allow to cool slightly.

5. Puree in a food processor or blender without adding extra fluid.

Asparagus Puree

10 asparagus spears, woody ends snapped off

1. Place a steamer basket in a pot and add enough water to just touch the bottom of the steamer basket.

2. Cover the pot and bring the water to a boil over high heat.

3. Add the asparagus, turn the heat down to medium, and loosely cover the pot.

4. Steam for 5 to 8 minutes, or until the asparagus is very soft. Allow to cool slightly.

5. Puree in a food processor or blender, adding breast milk or cooking water as needed to achieve the desired consistency.

Broccoli Puree

Florets from 1 head broccoli, cut into large pieces

1. Place a steamer basket in a pot and add enough water to just touch the bottom of the steamer basket.

2. Cover the pot and bring the water to a boil over high heat.

3. Add the broccoli, turn the heat down to medium, and loosely cover the pot.

4. Steam for 3 to 5 minutes, or until the broccoli is very soft. Allow to cool slightly.

5. Puree in a food processor or blender, adding breast milk or cooking water as needed to achieve the desired consistency.

Parsnip Puree

*1 parsnip, peeled
and cut into chunks*

1. Place a steamer basket in a pot and add enough water to just touch the bottom of the steamer basket.

2. Cover the pot and bring the water to a boil over high heat.

3. Add the parsnips, turn the heat down to medium, and loosely cover the pot.

4. Steam for 15 to 20 minutes, or until the parsnips are very soft. Allow to cool slightly.

5. Puree in a food processor or blender, adding breast milk or cooking water as needed to achieve the desired consistency.

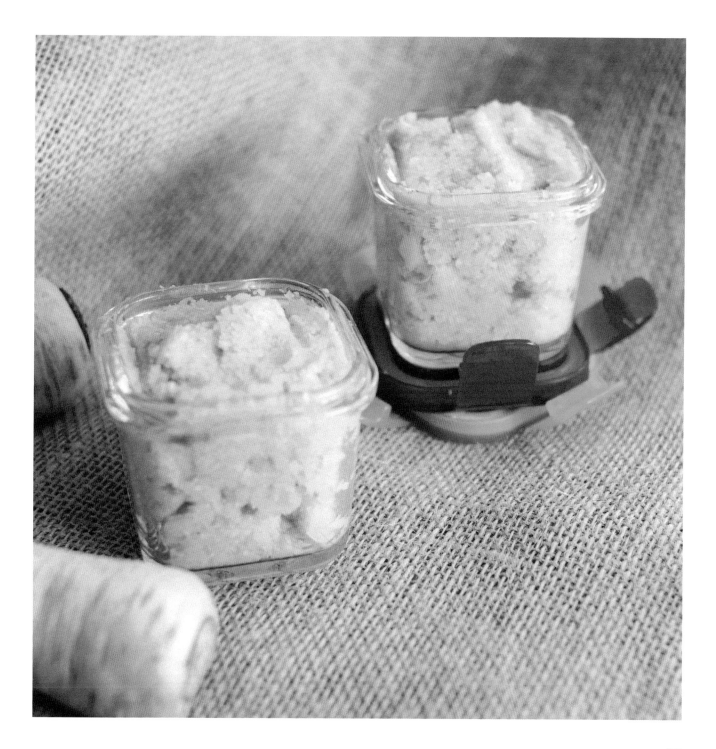

Cauliflower Puree

Florets from 1 head cauliflower, cut into large pieces

1. Place a steamer basket in a pot and add enough water to just touch the bottom of the steamer basket.

2. Cover the pot and bring the water to a boil over high heat.

3. Add the cauliflower, turn the heat down to medium, and loosely cover the pot.

4. Steam for 3 to 5 minutes, or until the cauliflower is very soft. Allow to cool slightly.

5. Puree in a food processor or blender, adding breast milk or cooking water as needed to achieve the desired consistency.

Eggplant Puree

1 large eggplant, peeled, seeded, and cut into chunks

1. Place a steamer basket in a pot and add enough water to just touch the bottom of the steamer basket.

2. Cover the pot and bring the water to a boil over high heat.

3. Add the eggplant, turn the heat down to medium, and loosely cover the pot.

4. Steam for 4 to 6 minutes, or until the eggplant is very soft. Allow to cool slightly.

5. Puree in a food processor or blender, adding breast milk or cooking water as needed to achieve the desired consistency.

Beet Puree

4 beets, peeled and cut into chunks

1. Place a steamer basket in a pot and add enough water to just touch the bottom of the steamer basket.

2. Cover the pot and bring the water to a boil over high heat.

3. Add the beets, turn the heat down to medium, and loosely cover the pot.

4. Steam for 40 to 50 minutes, or until the beets are very tender. Allow to cool slightly.

5. Puree in a food processor or blender, adding breast milk or cooking water as needed to achieve the desired consistency.

Cucumber Mush

1 cucumber, peeled and cut into chunks

1. Puree in a food processor or blender, adding breast milk or water as needed to achieve the desired consistency.

Corn Puree

2 ears corn,
husks and silk removed

1. Bring a large pot of water to a boil over high heat.

2. Place the corn in the boiling water and cover.

3. Cook for 10 minutes. Allow to cool slightly.

4. To cut the kernels from the cob, hold the stem of the corn and place the tip in the bottom of a large bowl. With a large chef's knife, use sawing motions down the cob, separating the kernels from the cob so that they fall into the bowl. (Or you can use a corn stripper tool designed for this purpose.)

5. Puree in a food processor or blender, adding breast milk or cooking water as needed to achieve the desired consistency.

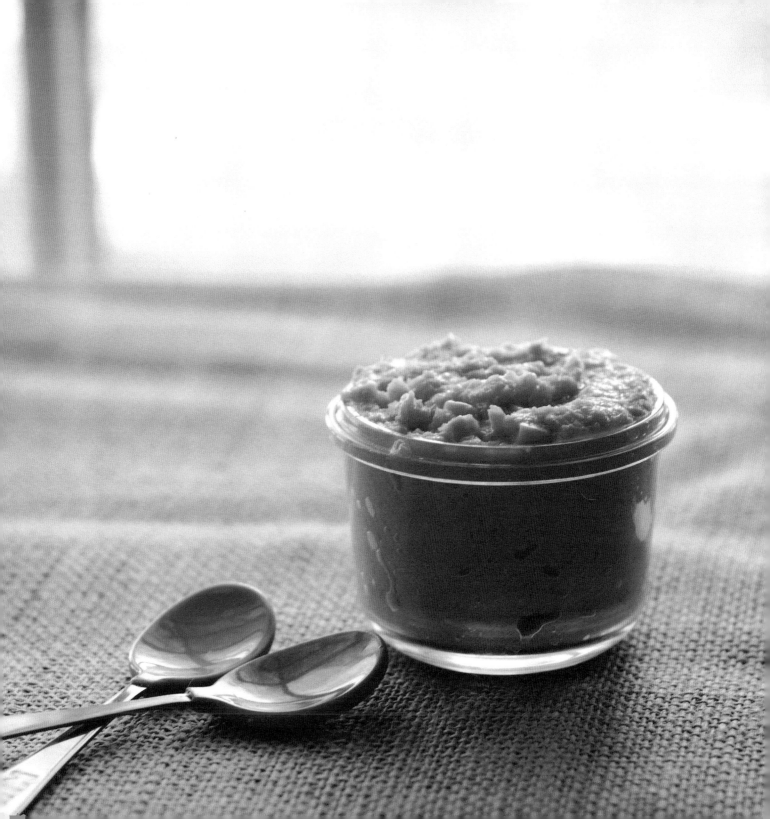

Spinach Puree

*1 bunch spinach,
woody stems removed*

1. Place a steamer basket in a pot and add enough water to just touch the bottom of the steamer basket.

2. Cover the pot and bring the water to a boil over high heat.

3. Add the spinach, turn the heat down to medium, and loosely cover the pot.

4. Steam for about 3 minutes, or until the spinach is wilted and very soft. Allow to cool slightly.

5. Puree in a food processor or blender, adding breast milk or cooking water as needed to achieve the desired consistency.

Tomato Puree

*3 large tomatoes,
cut into chunks*

1. Place a steamer basket in a pot and add enough water to just touch the bottom of the steamer basket.

2. Cover the pot and bring the water to a boil over high heat.

3. Add the tomatoes, turn the heat down to medium, and loosely cover the pot.

4. Steam for about 10 minutes, or until the tomatoes are very soft. Allow to cool slightly.

5. Puree in a food processor or blender, adding breast milk or cooking water as needed to achieve the desired consistency.

Artichoke Heart Puree

2 artichoke hearts,
canned with no salt or frozen
(If you can't find them, buy
2 artichokes and cut out the
hearts.)

1 lemon, halved

1. Bring a small pot of water to a boil over high heat.

2. Squeeze some lemon juice all over the artichoke hearts.

3. Squeeze some more lemon juice into the boiling water and add the artichoke hearts.

4. Turn the heat down to medium, loosely cover the pot, and boil for about 15 minutes, or until the artichoke hearts are soft.

5. Puree in a food processor or blender, adding breast milk or cooking water as needed to achieve the desired consistency.

Mashed White Potatoes

5 white potatoes, scrubbed

1. Preheat the oven to 400°F.

2. Poke the potatoes with a fork, seven times each.

3. Place the potatoes directly on the middle oven rack.

4. Bake for 45 minutes.

5. Allow to cool slightly. If this is a starter puree, remove the potato skin. If you want to add more texture and fiber, leave it on.

6. Puree in a food processor or blender, adding breast milk or water as needed to achieve the desired consistency.

Zucchini Puree

*1 zucchini, peeled
and cut into large pieces*

1. Place a steamer basket in a pot and add enough water to just touch the bottom of the steamer basket.

2. Cover the pot and bring the water to a boil over high heat.

3. Add the zucchini, turn the heat down to medium, and loosely cover the pot.

4. Steam for 3 to 5 minutes, or until the zucchini is very soft. Allow to cool slightly.

5. Puree in a food processor or blender, adding breast milk or cooking water as needed to achieve the desired consistency.

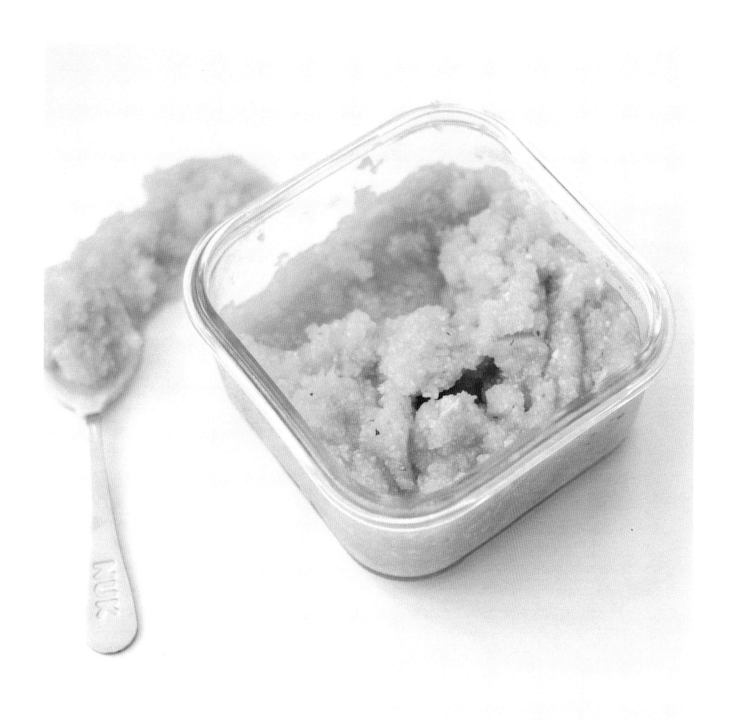

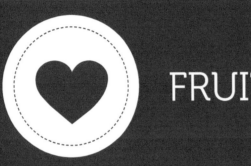

FRUIT PUREES

Plum Puree

5 plums, peeled, cut in half, pitted, and cut into chunks

1. Place a steamer basket in a pot and add enough water to just touch the bottom of the steamer basket.

2. Cover the pot and bring the water to a boil over high heat.

3. Add the plums, turn the heat down to medium, and loosely cover the pot.

4. Steam for 3 to 5 minutes, or until the plums are very soft. Allow to cool slightly.

5. Puree in a food processor or blender, adding breast milk or cooking water as needed to achieve the desired consistency.

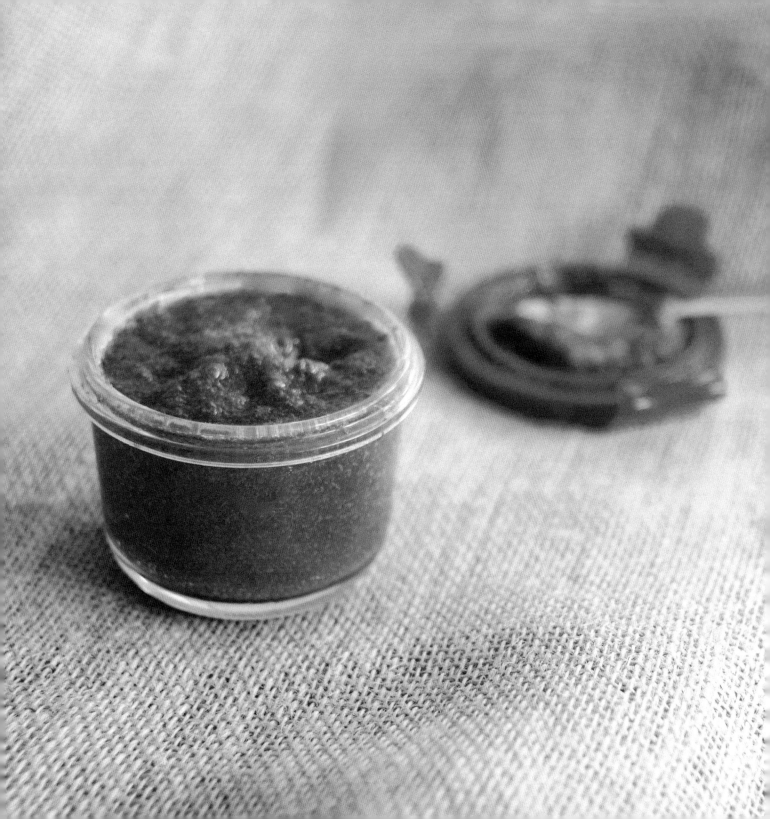

Avocado Mush

*1 avocado,
  peeled and pitted*

1. Place the avocado in a bowl and mash with your fork.

TIP: Avocado puree turns brown when frozen. The taste stays the same, but the texture will change. Our tip is to mash only half of the avocado, and freeze the other half still attached to the pit. Avocado stored in the fridge will also turn brown, so if your baby has leftovers you might want to finish them up yourself right away!

Roasted Apple Puree

*6 apples, peeled, cored,
  and cut into chunks*

1. Preheat the oven to 400°F.

2. Place the apples in a baking dish with just enough water to cover the bottom.

3. Bake for 30 minutes. Allow to cool slightly.

4. Puree in a food processor or blender, adding breast milk or water as needed to achieve the desired consistency.

Banana Mush

1 banana, peeled

1. Place the banana in a bowl and mash with your fork.

   TIP: Banana alone does not freeze well, nor store well after 2 days in the fridge. It is fine when mixed with other ingredients.

Pear Mush

6 very ripe pears

1. If this is a starter puree, peel the pears. If you want to add more texture and fiber, leave the peel on. Core the pears and cut into chunks.

2. Puree in a food processor or blender, adding breast milk or water as needed to achieve the desired consistency.

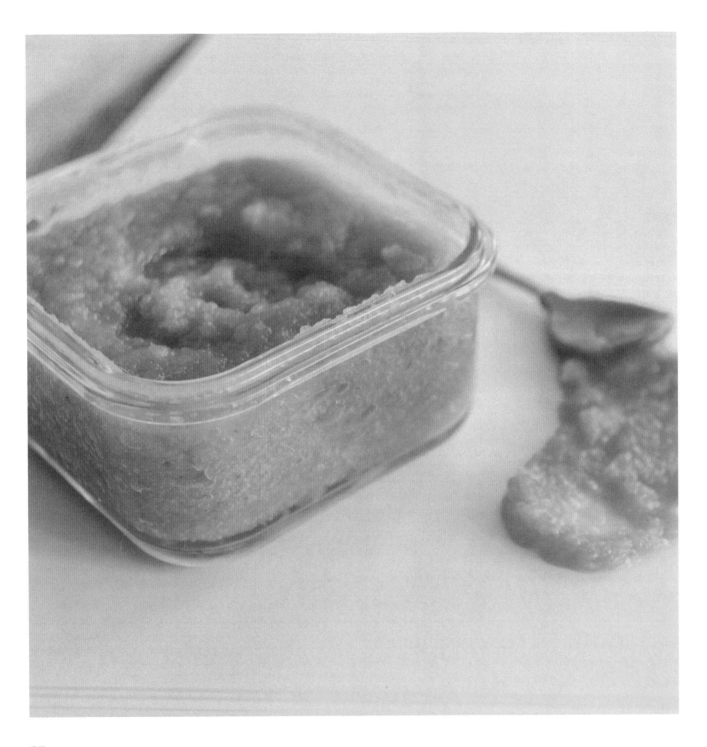

Cantaloupe Mush

1 large ripe cantaloupe, cut in half and seeded

1. Scoop out the cantaloupe from the peel.

2. Puree in a food processor or blender, adding breast milk or water as needed to achieve the desired consistency. Or dice into manageable pieces.

TIP: Cantaloupe puree does not freeze well. We suggest cutting the cantaloupe into small pieces and freezing them that way. If your weaner would rather have a puree, simply thaw the frozen pieces and then puree!

Roasted Apricot Puree

*6 medium apricots,
cut in half and pitted*

1. Preheat the oven to 400°F.

2. Place the apricots in a baking dish, cut sides down, with just enough water to cover the bottom.

3. Bake for 30 minutes.

4. Allow to cool slightly. Scoop out the apricots from the peel if this is a starter puree. If you want to add more texture and fiber, leave the peel on.

5. Puree in a food processor or blender, adding breast milk or water as needed to achieve the desired consistency.

Mango Puree

*1 mango, cut in half
lengthwise and pitted*

1. Place a steamer basket in a pot and add enough water to just touch the bottom of the steamer basket.

2. Cover the pot and bring the water to a boil over high heat.

3. Add the mango, turn the heat down to medium, and loosely cover the pot.

4. Steam for about 5 minutes, or until the mango is very soft. Allow to cool slightly.

5. Puree in a food processor or blender, adding breast milk or cooking water as needed to achieve the desired consistency.

Roasted Nectarine Puree

6 nectarines,
cut in half and pitted

1. Preheat the oven to 400°F.

2. Place the nectarines in a baking dish, cut sides down, with just enough water to cover the bottom.

3. Bake for 30 minutes.

4. Allow to cool slightly. Scoop out the nectarines from the peel if this is a starter puree. If you want to add more texture and fiber, leave the peel on.

5. Puree in a food processor or blender, adding breast milk or water as needed to achieve the desired consistency.

Roasted Peach Puree

6 peaches,
cut in half and pitted

1. Preheat the oven to 400°F.

2. Place the peaches in a baking dish, cut sides down, with just enough water to cover the bottom.

3. Bake for 30 minutes.

4. Allow to cool slightly. Scoop out the peaches from the peel if this is a starter puree. If you want to add more texture and fiber, leave the peel on.

5. Puree in a food processor or blender, adding breast milk or water as needed to achieve the desired consistency.

Cherry Puree

1 cup soft cherries, pitted

1. Puree in a food processor or blender, adding breast milk or water as needed to achieve the desired consistency.

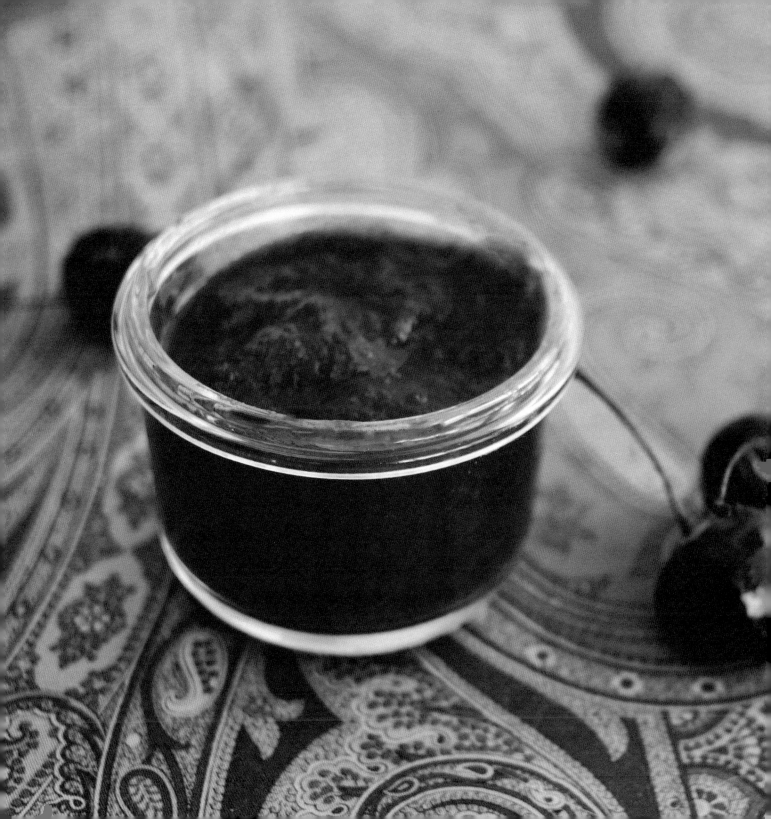

Persimmon Puree

5 persimmons,
peeled and diced

1. Place a steamer basket in a pot and add enough water to just touch the bottom of the steamer basket.

2. Cover the pot and bring the water to a boil over high heat.

3. Add the persimmons, turn the heat down to medium, and loosely cover the pot.

4. Steam for 5 to 7 minutes, or until the persimmons are very soft. Allow to cool slightly.

5. Puree in a food processor or blender, adding breast milk or cooking water as needed to achieve the desired consistency.

Prune Puree

12 prunes (dried plums)

1. Place a steamer basket in a pot and add enough water to just touch the bottom of the steamer basket.

2. Cover the pot and bring the water to a boil over high heat.

3. Add the prunes, turn the heat down to medium, and loosely cover the pot.

4. Steam for 5 minutes, or until the prunes are very soft. Allow to cool slightly.

5. Puree in a food processor or blender, adding breast milk or cooking water as needed to achieve the desired consistency.

Melon Puree

1 large ripe melon,
cut in half and seeded

1. Scoop out the melon from the peel.

2. Puree in a food processor or blender, adding breast milk or water as needed to achieve the desired consistency.

TIP: Melon puree does not freeze well. We suggest cutting the melon into small pieces and freezing them that way. If your weaner would rather have a puree, simply thaw the frozen pieces and then puree!

Blueberry Puree

1 cup blueberries

1. Puree in a food processor or blender, adding breast milk or water as needed to achieve the desired consistency.

Papaya Mush

1 large ripe papaya,
peeled and seeded

1. Puree in a food processor or blender, adding breast milk or water as needed to achieve the desired consistency.

TIP: With a very ripe papaya, you can even skip the pureeing step and just mash the papaya with a fork.

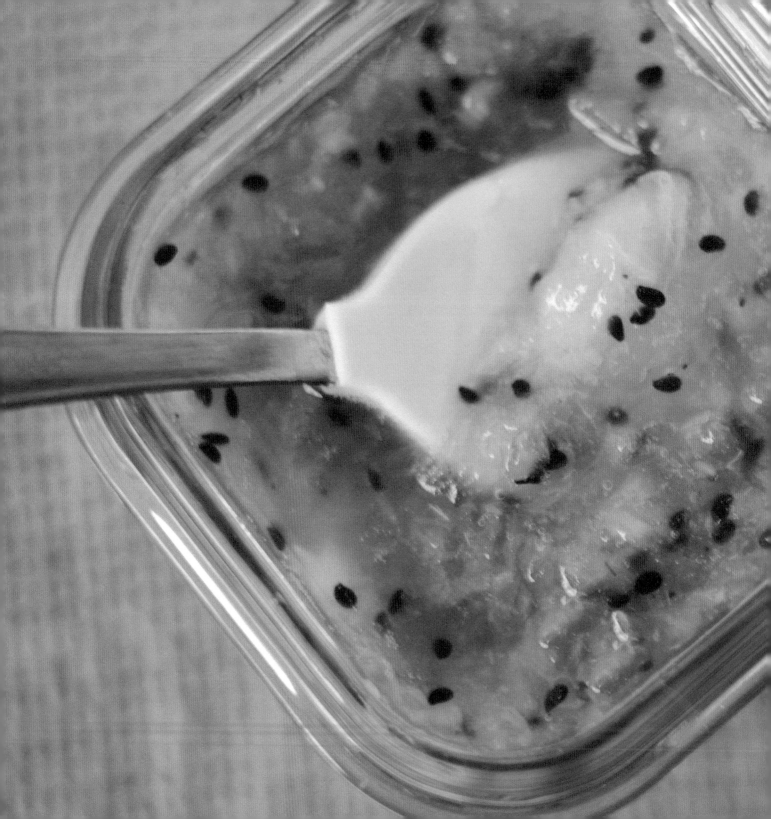

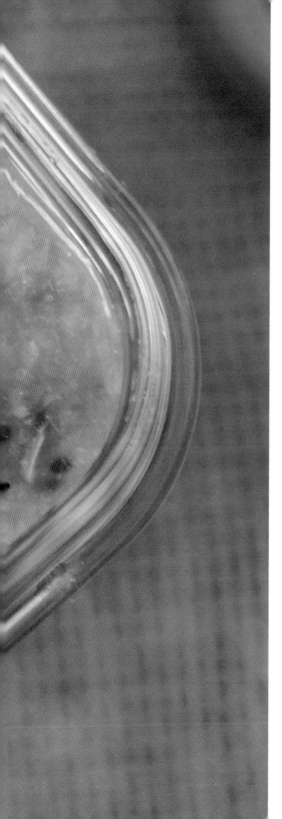

Kiwi Mush

1 large kiwi, peeled

1. Puree in a food processor or blender, adding breast milk or water as needed to achieve the desired consistency.

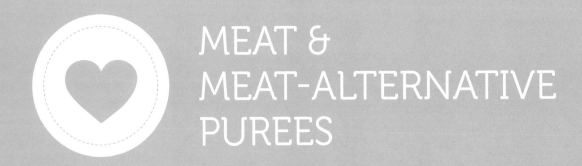

MEAT &
MEAT-ALTERNATIVE
PUREES

Dried Bean Puree

1 cup dried beans

You can use black beans, chickpeas, Great Northern beans, lima beans (large or baby), navy or small white beans, pink beans, pinto beans, red beans, red kidney beans, or soybeans, but do not mix different types of beans in the same batch.

1. Place the beans in a medium-size pot and add enough water to cover. Cover the pot and allow the beans to soak overnight.

2. Drain the beans and then return them to the pot. Add enough fresh water to cover.

3. Bring the water to a boil over high heat.

4. Reduce the heat to low, cover the pot, and simmer until the beans are tender.
   Lima beans (large): **1 hour**
   Lima beans (baby): **50 minutes**
   Black beans, garbanzo beans, Great Northern beans, navy or small white beans, pink beans, pinto beans, red beans, red kidney beans: **1 hour and 15 minutes**
   Soybeans: **3 hours**

5. Drain the cooked beans and then puree in a food processor or blender, adding breast milk or cooking water as needed to achieve the desired consistency.

TIP: Cooked beans are also a great starter finger food, if your weaner is interested in feeding him- or herself! For larger beans, just gently mash a cooked bean with your finger, or cut it in half to prevent choking.

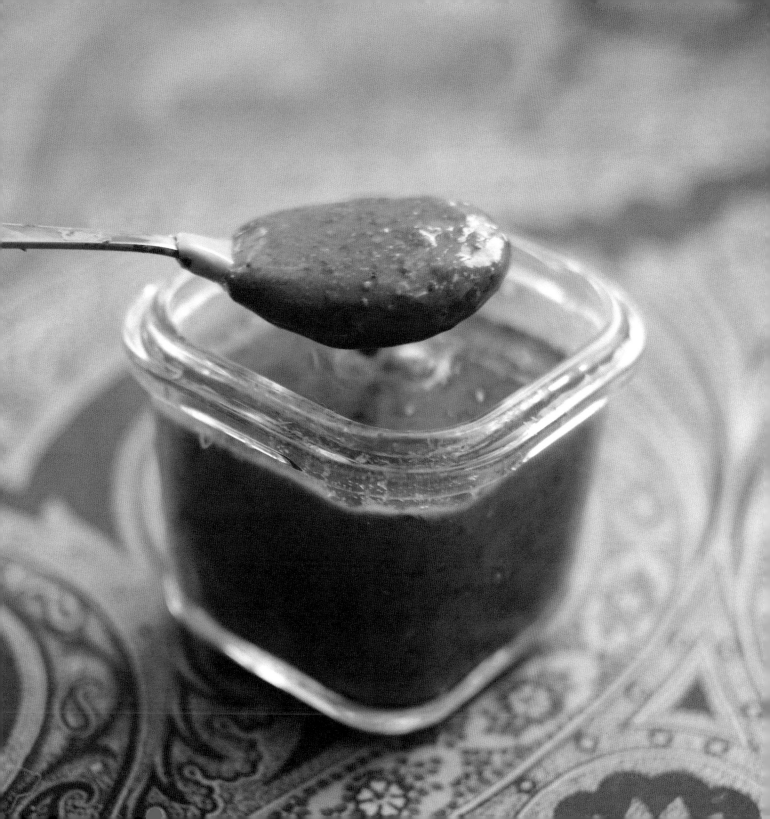

Dried Bean Puree NOT SOAKED

1 cup dried beans

This recipe requires no overnight soaking. You can use black-eyed peas, green split peas, or lentils, but do not mix different types of beans in the same batch.

1. Place the beans in a medium-size pot and add enough water to cover.

2. Bring the water to a boil over high heat.

3. Reduce the heat to low, cover the pot, and simmer until the beans are tender.

4. Green split peas and lentils: **30 minutes**

5. Black-eyed peas: **1 hour and 15 minutes**

6. Drain the cooked beans and then puree in a food processor or blender, adding breast milk or cooking water as needed to achieve the desired consistency.

TIP: Cooked beans are also a great starter finger food, if your weaner is interested in feeding him- or herself! For larger beans, just gently mash a cooked bean with your finger, or cut it in half to prevent choking.

Egg Yolk

1 egg yolk

1. Fry the egg yolk in a small nonstick skillet over medium heat, stirring for about 2 minutes, or until fully cooked.

2. Allow to cool slightly, and then mash with a fork

3. Serve immediately, as egg yolk does not keep well in the refrigerator or freezer.

Tofu Mush

1 package silken tofu, drained

1. Mash with a fork.

NOTE: Once your weaner is ready for finger foods, you can buy firm tofu and grate it!

Beefy baby or Bison Puree

*1 pound extra-lean ground
beef or ground bison*

1. Fry the beef or bison in a large skillet over medium high heat, breaking up the chunks and stirring occasionally for about 10 minutes, until there is no pink left.

2. Transfer the cooked meat to a few layers of paper towels to drain off any fat. Allow to cool slightly.

3. Puree in a food processor or blender, adding breast milk or water as needed to achieve the desired consistency.

TIP: You can use any ground meat for this recipe, including chicken and turkey, too.

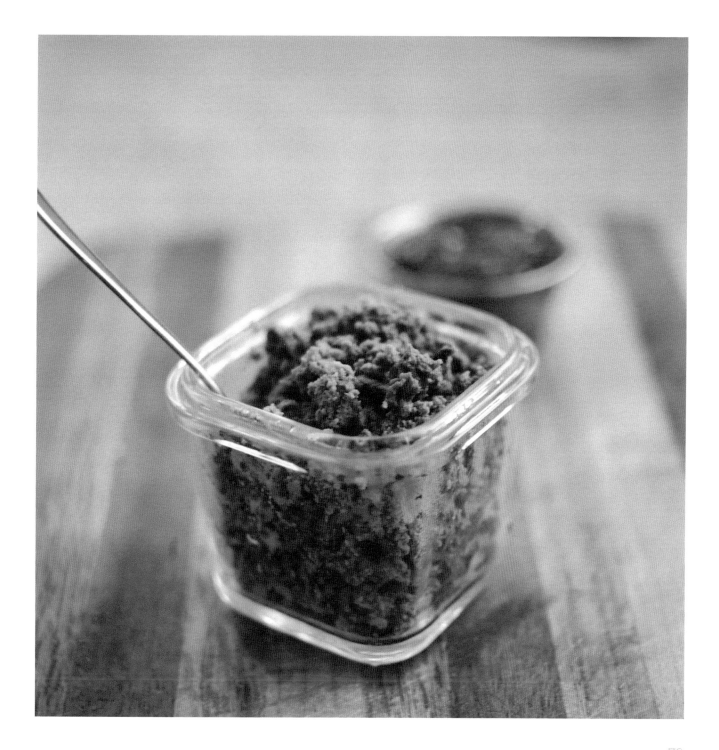

Beefy baby or Bison Puree

*1 pound extra-lean ground
beef or ground bison*

1. Bring a large pot of water to a boil over high heat.

2. Add the ground beef or bison and continue to boil for about 20 minutes, or until there is no pink left.

3. Drain the cooked meat in a colander and allow to cool slightly.

4. Puree in a food processor or blender, adding breast milk or water as needed to achieve the desired consistency.

TIP: You can use any ground meat for this recipe, including chicken and turkey, too. And you can boil any of the meat recipes instead of frying or baking, if you prefer. While messy, boiling adds some moisture to the meat, making it a bit easier to puree.

Pork Tenderloin Puree

½ pound pork tenderloin

1. Preheat the oven to 325°F.

2. Place the pork in a baking pan.

3. Insert a meat thermometer into the center of the tenderloin.

4. Cook for about 35 minutes, or until the meat thermometer reads 160°F.

5. Allow to cool slightly, and then cut the pork into chunks.

6. Puree in a food processor or blender, adding breast milk or water as needed to achieve the desired consistency.

Chicken Puree

2 boneless, skinless chicken breasts or thighs (Dark meat is moister and has more iron!)

1. Preheat the oven to 375°F.

2. Place the chicken pieces in a baking pan and bake for 20 to 40 minutes (shorter for breasts, longer for thighs), until a meat thermometer reads 155°F for breasts and 180°F for thighs.

3. Allow to cool slightly, and then cut the chicken into large chunks.

4. Puree in a food processor or blender, adding breast milk or water as needed to achieve the desired consistency.

Top Sirloin Roast Puree

1 pound top sirloin roast

1. Preheat the oven to 325°F.

2. Place the roast in a baking pan, fat side up.

3. Insert a meat thermometer into the center of the roast.

4. Cook for about 30 minutes, or until the meat thermometer reads 160°F.

5. Allow to cool slightly, trim off any visible fat, and cut the roast into chunks.

6. Puree in a food processor or blender, adding breast milk or water as needed to achieve the desired consistency.

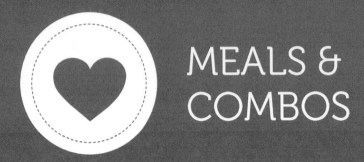

MEALS & COMBOS

Apple Oatmeal

1¼ cups water

½ cup homemade
   oatmeal powder
   (see Cereal Powder recipe on page 19)

5 apples, peeled, cored,
   and diced

1. Place the water in a large pot and bring to a boil over high heat.

2. Using your whisk, stir in the rice powder and the apples.

3. Turn the heat down to medium and whisk constantly for 10 minutes.

4. This may be a good texture for your weaner. Or, if needed, cool slightly and then puree in a food processor or blender, adding breast milk or water as needed to achieve the desired consistency.

TIP: It's easy to spice up breakfast. Take any of your weaner's favorite fruit purees and add it to their cereal. They do not have to be cooked at the same time. If you are making a fresh batch of cereal, you can always thaw a fruit Wean Cube and throw it in with the cereal.

Purple Barley Plum Cereal

1¼ cups water

½ cup homemade barley powder

(see Cereal Powder recipe on page 19)

5 plums, pitted, peeled, and diced

1. Place the water in a large pot and bring to a boil over high heat.

2. Using your whisk, stir in the barley powder and the plums.

3. Turn the heat down to medium and whisk constantly for 10 minutes.

4. This may be a good texture for your weaner. Or, if needed, cool slightly and then puree in a food processor or blender, adding breast milk or water as needed to achieve the desired consistency.

Figs 'n' Oat Breakfast

1½ cups water

½ cup homemade oatmeal powder

(see Cereal Powder recipe on page 19)

1 cup chopped dried figs

2 Wean Cubes (1 cup) applesauce

1. Place the water in a large pot and bring to a boil over high heat.

2. Using your whisk, stir in the oatmeal powder and the figs.

3. Turn the heat down to medium and whisk constantly for 10 minutes.

4. Add applesauce into your mix.

5. This may be a good texture for your weaner. Or, if needed, cool slightly and then puree in a food processor or blender, adding breast milk or water as needed to achieve the desired consistency.

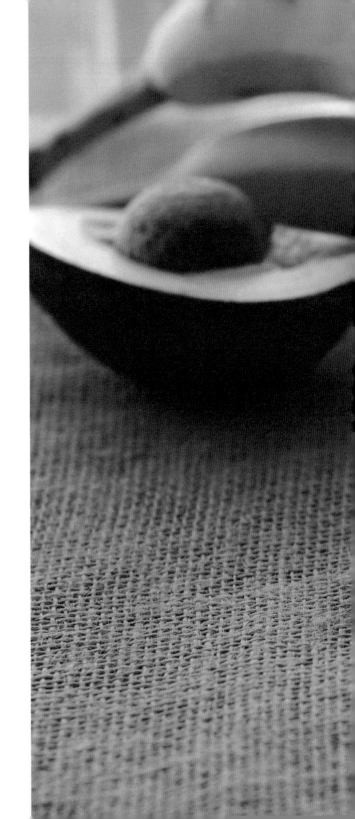

Quick and Easy Bananacado

1 avocado, peeled and pitted

1 banana, peeled

1. Puree the banana and avocado in a food processor or blender, adding breast milk or water as needed to achieve the desired consistency. Or, if the avocado and banana are very ripe, you can just mash them with a fork, leaving some chunks for your weaner to try some new textures!

TIP: If frozen, the bananacado turns a bit brown but still tastes great.

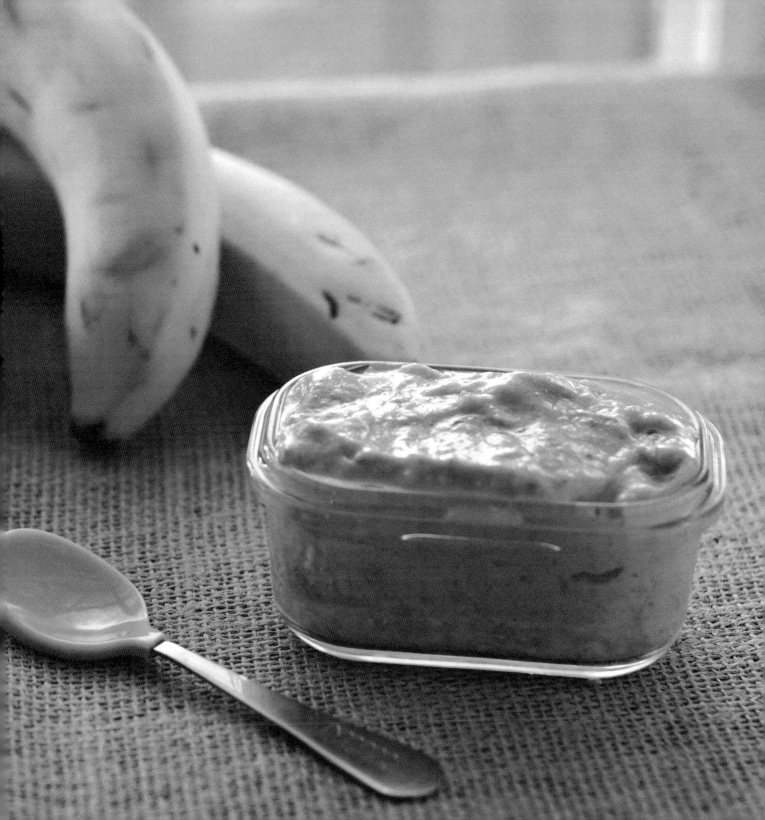

Pear and Apple Mix

*3 apples, peeled, cored, and
cut into chunks*

*3 pears, peeled, cored, and
cut into chunks*

1. Place a steamer basket in a pot and add enough water to just
touch the bottom of the steamer basket.

2. Cover the pot and bring the water to a boil over high heat.

3. Add the apples and pears, turn the heat down to medium, and
loosely cover the pot.

4. Steam for about 10 minutes, or until the fruit is very tender.
Allow to cool slightly.

5. Puree in a food processor or blender, adding breast milk or
cooking water as needed to achieve the desired consistency.

Brown Rice and Green Peas

1¼ cups water

*½ cup homemade
brown rice powder*
(see Cereal Powder recipe on page 19)

1 cup peas, fresh or frozen

1. Place the water in a large pot and bring to a boil over high heat.

2. Using your whisk, stir in the rice powder and the peas.

3. Turn the heat down to medium and whisk constantly for 10
minutes.

This should be a great texture for your weaner, as is!

TIP: Remember that oat, barley, and rice cereal are not just for
breakfast—you can mix in any fruit or veggie with the cereals to
make a filling lunch or supper!

Steamed Peas and Carrots

10 carrots, peeled and cut into chunks

2 cups peas, fresh or frozen

1. Place a steamer basket in a pot and add enough water to just touch the bottom of the steamer basket.

2. Cover the pot and bring the water to a boil over high heat.

3. Add the carrots, turn the heat down to medium, and loosely cover the pot.

4. Steam for 5 minutes, add the peas, and loosely cover the pot again.

5. Steam for another 5 minutes, or until the veggies are very soft. Allow to cool slightly.

6. Puree the peas and carrots together in a food processor or blender, adding breast milk or cooking water as needed to achieve the desired consistency.

Peaches and Bananas

6 peaches, cut in half and pitted

2 bananas, peeled

1. Preheat the oven to 400°F.

2. Place the peaches in a baking dish, cut sides down, with just enough water to cover the bottom.

3. Bake for 30 minutes.

4. Scoop out the peaches from the peel if this is a starter puree. If you want to add more texture and fiber, leave the peel on.

5. Puree the peaches and bananas together in a food processor or blender, adding breast milk or water as needed to achieve the desired consistency.

Tummy Delight Prunes and Brown Rice

1¼ cups water

½ cup homemade
   brown rice powder
   (see Cereal Powder recipe on page 19)

12 prunes (dried plums)

1. Place the water in a large pot and bring to a boil over high heat.

2. Using your whisk, stir in the rice powder and prunes.

3. Turn the heat down to medium and whisk constantly for 10 minutes. Allow to cool slightly.

4. Puree in a food processor or blender, adding breast milk or water as needed to achieve the desired consistency.

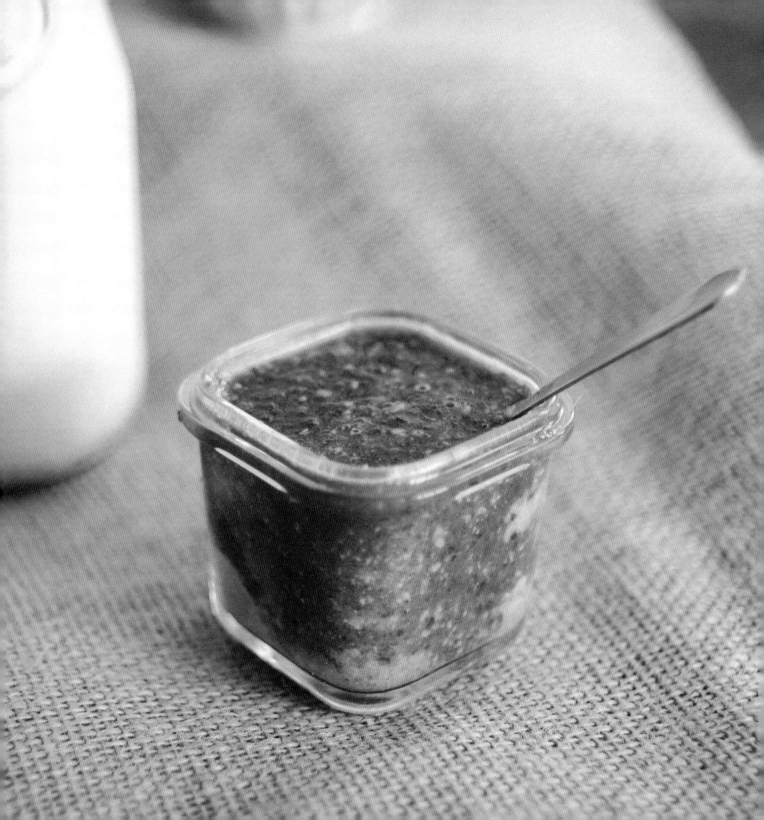

Green Beans and Pears

*1 pound green beans,
ends trimmed*

*5 pears, peeled (if desired)
and cored*

1. Place a steamer basket in a pot and add enough water to just touch the bottom of the steamer basket.

2. Cover the pot and bring the water to a boil over high heat.

3. Add the green beans and pears, turn the heat down to medium, and loosely cover the pot.

4. Steam for about 15 minutes, or until the beans and pears are very tender. Allow to cool slightly.

5. Puree the green beans and pears together in a food processor or blender, adding breast milk or cooking water as needed to achieve the desired consistency.

Pumpkin and Carrot Mush

*1 pumpkin, cut in half
and gutted*

*10 carrots, peeled and
cut into chunks*

1. Preheat the oven to 400°F.

2. Put the pumpkin in a baking pan, cut sides down. Add the carrots and just enough water to cover the bottom.

3. Bake for 45 minutes.

4. Allow to cool slightly. Scoop out the pumpkin from the skin.

5. Puree the pumpkin and carrots together in a food processor or blender, adding breast milk or water as needed to achieve the desired consistency.

Sweet Potatoes and Green Beans

1 pound green beans, ends trimmed

5 sweet potatoes, peeled and cut into chunks

1. Preheat the oven to 400°F.

2. Place the sweet potatoes and green beans in a casserole dish with just enough water to cover the bottom.

3. Bake for 1 hour. Allow to cool slightly.

4. Puree the sweet potatoes and green beans together in a food processor or blender, adding breast milk or water as needed to achieve the desired consistency.

Yellow Squash and Apples

1 yellow squash, cut in half lengthwise and seeded

5 apples, cored and cut into chunks (keep peel on, for texture)

1. Preheat the oven to 400°F.

2. Put the squash in a baking pan, cut sides down. Add the apples and just enough water to cover the bottom.

3. Bake for 45 minutes. Allow to cool slightly.

4. Scoop out the squash from the peel.

5. Puree the squash and apples together in a food processor or blender, adding breast milk or water as needed to achieve the desired consistency.

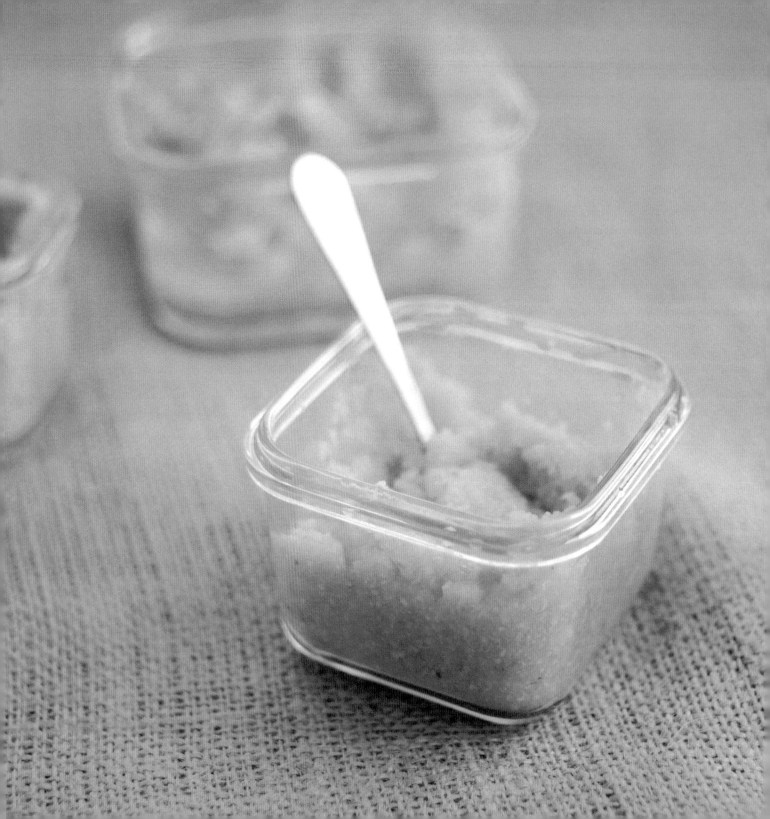

Parsnips and Zucchini

*1 parsnip, peeled and cut
   into chunks*

*1 zucchini, peeled and
   cut into chunks*

1. Place a steamer basket in a pot and add enough water to just touch the bottom of the steamer basket.

2. Cover the pot and bring the water to a boil over high heat.

3. Add the parsnips, turn the heat down to medium, and loosely cover the pot.

4. Steam for 13 minutes, add the zucchini, and loosely cover the pot again.

5. Steam for an additional 5 minutes. Allow to cool slightly.

6. Puree the parsnips and zucchini together in a food processor or blender, adding breast milk or cooking water as needed to achieve the desired consistency.

Sweet Potatoes and Pumpkin

5 sweet potatoes

*1 pumpkin, cut in half
and gutted*

1. Preheat the oven to 400°F.

2. Put the pumpkin in the baking pan, cut sides down, with just
   enough water to cover the bottom.

3. Poke the sweet potatoes with a fork, seven times each. Wrap
   each sweet potato in foil and place either in the baking pan
   with the pumpkin or directly on the middle oven rack.

4. Bake for 1 hour.

5. Allow to cool slightly. Scoop out the pumpkin from the peel.
   Unwrap the sweet potatoes, cut them in half, and then pull off
   the skins.

6. Puree the pumpkin and sweet potatoes together in a food
   processor or blender, adding breast milk or water as needed to
   achieve the desired consistency.

Mangos and Apricots

*5 mangos, cut in half
lengthwise and pitted*

*5 apricots, cut in half
and pitted*

1. Preheat the oven to 400°F.

2. Place the mangos and the apricots in a baking pan, cut sides
   down, with just enough water to cover the bottom.

3. Bake for 30 minutes. Allow to cool slightly.

4. Scoop out the fruit from the peels.

5. Puree the mangos and apricots together in a food processor or
   blender, adding breast milk or water as needed to achieve the
   desired consistency.

Pork and Apple

½ pound pork tenderloin

5 apples, peeled (if desired), cored, and cut into chunks

½ medium onion, cut into chunks

5 small turnips, peeled and cut into chunks

1. Preheat the oven to 325°F.

2. Place the pork in a lightly greased baking pan and add the apples and veggies around it.

3. Insert a meat thermometer into the center of the tenderloin.

4. Cook for 35 minutes or until the meat thermometer reads 160°F.

5. Dice the pork, apples, and veggies into small pieces or puree them together in a food processor or blender, adding breast milk or water as needed to achieve the desired consistency.

Blueberry Melon Head

1 fresh melon, cut in half and seeded

1 cup blueberries

1. Scoop out the melon from the peel.

2. Dice the melon and blueberries into small pieces or puree them together in a food processor or blender, adding breast milk or water as needed to achieve the desired consistency.

TIP: Melon puree does not freeze well. We suggest cutting the melon into small pieces and freezing them that way. If your weaner would rather have a puree, simply thaw the frozen pieces and then puree!

Sweet Apple Potatoes

2 sweet potatoes, peeled
and cut into chunks

3 apples, cored and cut
into chunks (keep peel on,
for texture)

1. Preheat the oven to 400°F.

2. Place the sweet potatoes and apples in a casserole
   dish with just enough water to cover the bottom.

3. Bake for 45 minutes.

4. Puree the sweet potatoes and apples together in a
   food processor or blender, adding breast milk or water
   as needed to achieve the desired consistency.

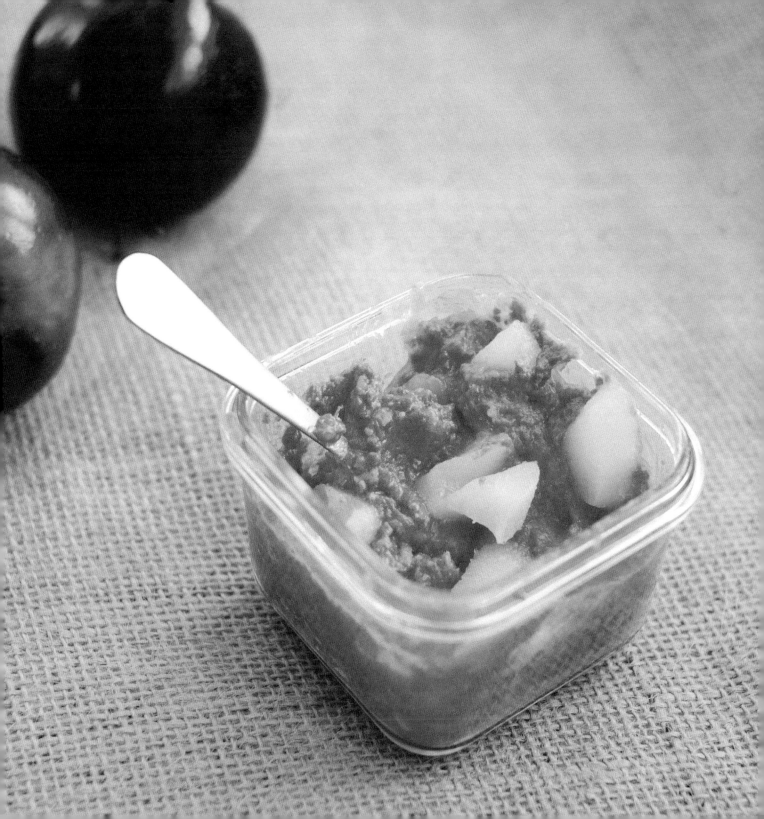

Acorn Squash and Nectarines

1 acorn squash, cut in half and seeded

5 nectarines, cut in half and pitted

1. Preheat oven to 400°F.

2. Put the squash and nectarines in a baking pan, cut sides down, with just enough water to cover the bottom.

3. Bake for 45 minutes.

4. Allow to cool slightly. Scoop out the squash from the skin and the nectarine from the peels (or keep the nectarine peels on, if desired, for more texture).

5. Puree the squash and nectarines together in a food processor or blender, adding breast milk or water as needed to achieve the desired consistency.

Tofu Banana Wheat Germ

1 package silken tofu

1 banana, peeled

1 tablespoon wheat germ

1. Dice the tofu and banana into small pieces and roll them in the wheat germ. Or puree the ingredients together in a food processor or blender, adding breast milk or water as needed to achieve the desired consistency.

Fruit Salad

1 cantaloupe, cut in half
  and seeded

1 cup seedless grapes, peeled

1 cup blueberries

1. Scoop out the cantaloupe from the peel, and add to the grapes and blueberries.

2. Dice the fruit into small pieces or puree them together in a food processor or blender, adding breast milk or water as needed to achieve the desired consistency.

Sweet Chicken

4 sweet potatoes

2 boneless, skinless
  chicken breasts

1. Preheat the oven to 400°F.

2. Poke the sweet potatoes with a fork, seven times each. Wrap each sweet potato in foil and place directly on the middle oven rack. Bake for 40 minutes.

3. Place the chicken in a baking pan. Bake the sweet potatoes and chicken for another 20 minutes.

4. Allow to cool slightly. Unwrap the sweet potatoes, cut them in half, and then pull off the skins.

5. Dice the sweet potatoes and chicken into small pieces, or puree them together in a food processor or blender, adding breast milk or water as needed to achieve the desired consistency.

Butternut Squashed Carrots

10 carrots, peeled and sliced

*1 medium butternut squash,
 cut in half lengthwise and seeded*

1. Preheat the oven to 400°F.

2. Put the squash in a baking pan, cut sides down. Add the carrots and just enough water to cover the bottom.

3. Bake for 45 minutes.

4. Allow to cool slightly. Scoop out the squash from the skin.

5. Puree the squash and carrots together in a food processor or blender, adding breast milk or water as needed to achieve the desired consistency.

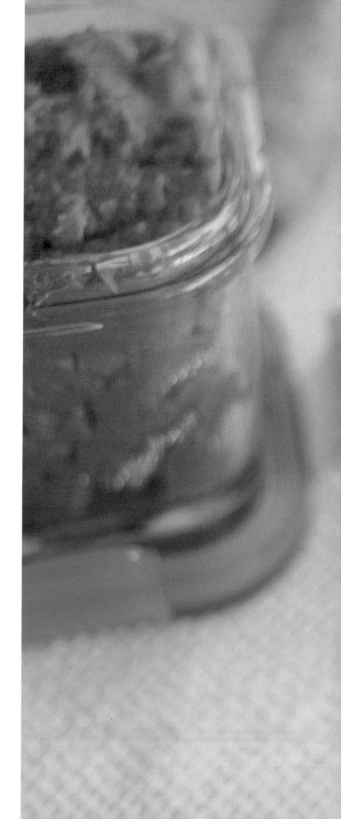

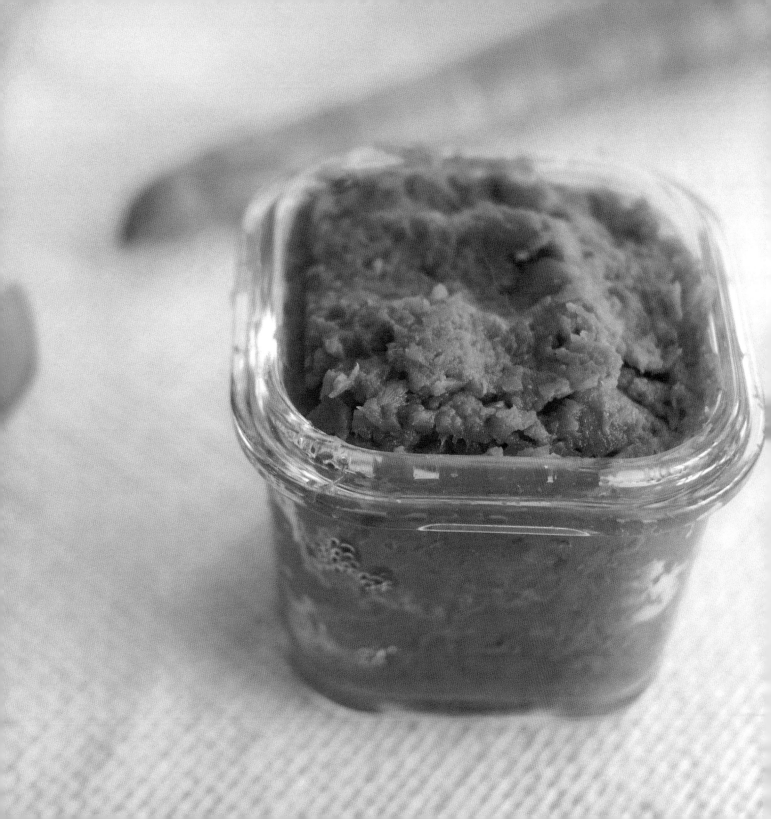

Baked Chicken and Carrots

*2 boneless, skinless
chicken breasts*

*10 carrots, peeled and
cut into chunks*

1. Preheat the oven to 400°F.

2. Place the chicken and carrots in a casserole dish with just enough water to cover the bottom.

3. Bake for 25 minutes. Allow to cool slightly.

4. Dice the chicken and carrots into small pieces or puree them together in a food processor or blender, adding breast milk or water as needed to achieve the desired consistency.

Basic Veggies

*4 white potatoes,
scrubbed or peeled,
and cut into chunks*

*10 carrots, peeled and
cut into chunks*

1 cup peas, fresh or frozen

1. Preheat the oven to 400°F.

2. Combine the veggies in a baking dish with just enough water to cover the bottom.

3. Bake for 45 minutes. Allow to cool slightly.

4. Dice the veggies into small pieces or puree them together in a food processor or blender, adding breast milk or water as needed to achieve the desired consistency.

Turnip Beet Mix

5 beets, peeled and cut into chunks

2 large turnips, peeled and cut into chunks

1. Place a steamer basket in a pot and add enough water to just touch the bottom of the steamer basket.

2. Cover the pot and bring the water to a boil over high heat.

3. Add the beets and turnips, turn the heat down to medium, and loosely cover the pot.

4. Steam for 40 to 50 minutes, or until the veggies are very tender. Allow to cool slightly.

5. Dice the beets and turnips into small pieces or puree them together in a food processor or blender, adding breast milk or water as needed to achieve the desired consistency.

Peppery Eggplant

1 teaspoon extra-virgin olive oil

1 eggplant, peeled, seeded, and cut into chunks

1 large red pepper, seeded and cut into chunks

1. Heat the oil in a large skillet over medium-high heat.

2. Add the eggplant and pepper and sauté for about 10 minutes, or until soft.

3. Dice the eggplant and pepper into small pieces or puree them together in a food processor or blender, adding breast milk or water as needed to achieve the desired consistency.

Smashed Baby Burgers

1 pound extra-lean ground beef

½ cup homemade bread crumbs
(see recipe below)

1. Preheat the oven to 400°F.

2. Mix the ground beef and breadcrumbs together with your hands and place in a lightly greased loaf pan.

3. Bake for 45 minutes. Allow to cool slightly.

4. Dice into small pieces.

Bread Crumbs

*10 slices whole-grain
bread, cubed*

1. Preheat the oven to 225°F.

2. Place the bread on a baking sheet.

3. Bake for 5 minutes, turn the bread over, and continue baking for another 5 minutes.

4. Allow the bread to cool completely and then grind it in your food processor.

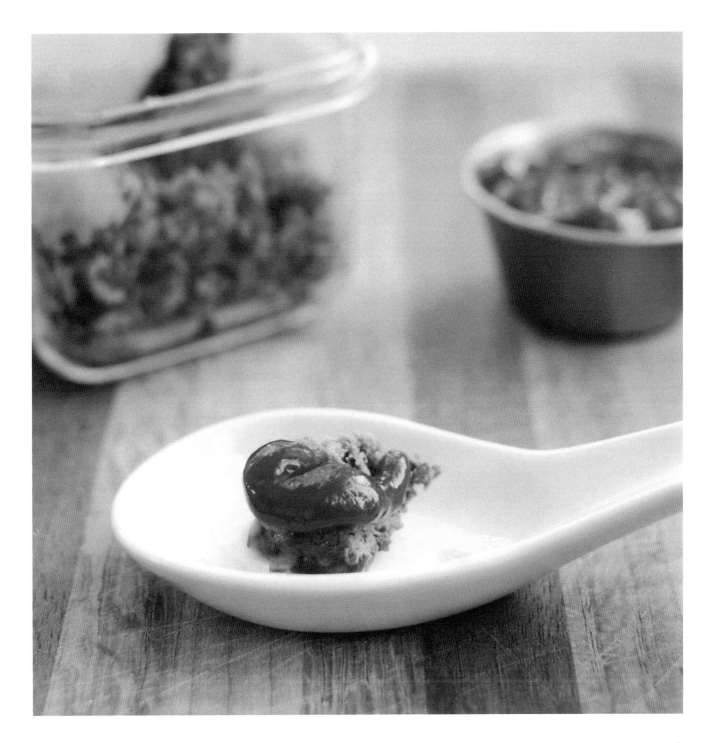

A Cherry Date

1 cup cherries, pitted

1 cup pitted dried dates

1. Dice the cherries and dates into small pieces or puree them together in a food processor or blender, adding breast milk or water as needed to achieve the desired consistency.

Papaya Banana Combomba

1 papaya, peeled, cut in half lengthwise, and seeded

1 banana, peeled

1. Dice the papaya and banana into small pieces or puree them together in a food processor or blender, adding breast milk or water as needed to achieve the desired consistency.

Green Potatoes

5 white potatoes, peeled and cut into chunks

5 asparagus spears, woody ends snapped off

1. Preheat the oven to 400°F.

2. Place the potatoes in a baking dish and bake for 30 minutes.

3. Add the asparagus to the pan, and bake with the potatoes for another 15 minutes.

4. Dice the potatoes and asparagus into small pieces or puree them together in a food processor or blender, adding breast milk or water as needed to achieve the desired consistency.

Zucchini and Apples

1 large zucchini, cut into chunks

5 apples, peeled (if desired), cored, and cut into chunks

1 teaspoon ground cinnamon

1. Place a steamer basket in a pot and add enough water to just touch the bottom of the steamer basket.

2. Cover the pot and bring the water to a boil over high heat.

3. Add the zucchini and apples, turn the heat down to medium, and loosely cover the pot.

4. Steam for 3 to 5 minutes, or until the zucchini and apples are very tender.

5. Transfer the apples and zucchini to a bowl and stir in the cinnamon.

6. Dice the apples and zucchini into small pieces or puree them together in a food processor or blender, adding breast milk or water as needed to achieve the desired consistency.

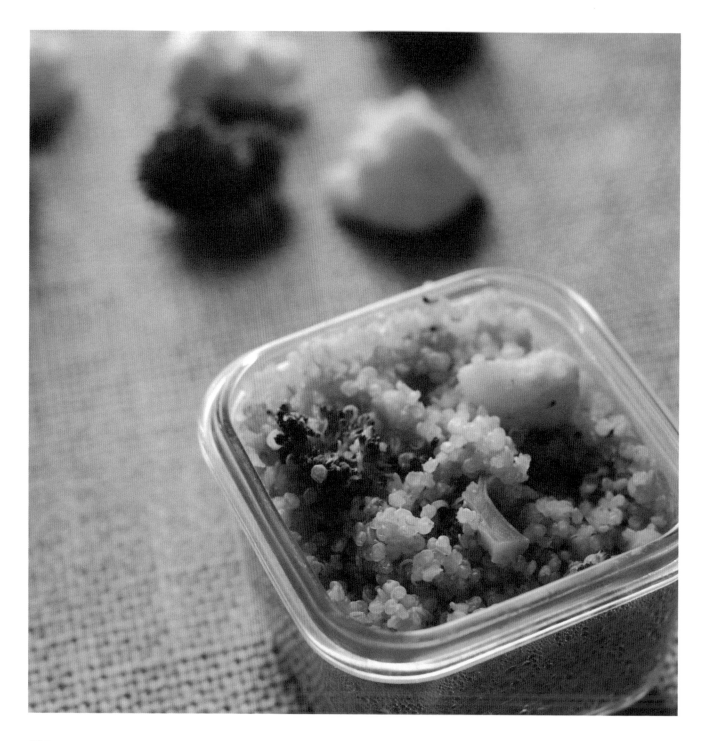

Quinoa and Veggies

1¾ cups water

½ cup uncooked quinoa

Florets from ¼ head broccoli,
cut into pieces

Florets from ¼ head cauliflower,
cut into pieces

1. Bring the water to a boil in a large pot over high heat.

2. Add the quinoa, broccoli, and cauliflower. Cover the pot and turn the heat to low.

3. Simmer for 15 minutes or until the quinoa opens up (like popcorn).

4. Dice the quinoa and veggies into small pieces or puree them together in a food processor or blender, adding breast milk or water as needed to achieve the desired consistency.

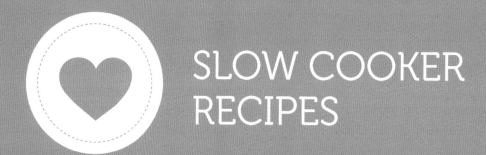

SLOW COOKER RECIPES

Slow cooking rocks a tired mama's world! Here are some easy recipes that don't require a lot of maintenance. These meals are bland enough for weaners yet tasty enough for all!

Slow Cooker Applesauce

8–10 apples, peeled, cored,
and chopped

½ cup water

1 teaspoon cinnamon
(optional)

1. Combine all ingredients in the slow cooker and stir.

2. Cover and cook on high for 4 to 6 hours.

3. This may be a perfect texture for your weaner, or you can puree in a food processor or blender, adding breast milk or water as needed to achieve the desired consistency.

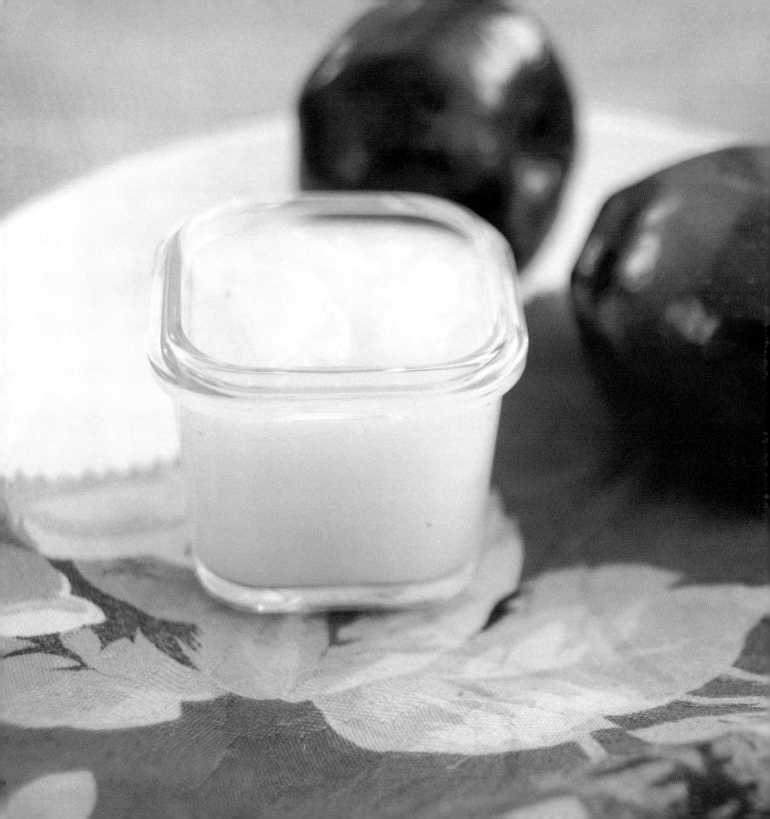

Slow Cooker Brown Rice

1 cup uncooked
   short-grain brown rice

1 teaspoon wheat germ

5½ cups water

1. Combine all ingredients in the slow cooker and stir.

2. Cover and cook on low for 6 to 8 hours.

3. This should be a great texture for your weaner, or you can puree in a food processor or blender, adding breast milk or water as needed to achieve the desired consistency.

Slow Cooker Kamut Blueberry Breakfast

1 cup uncooked Kamut

3 cups water

2 cups blueberries

½ cup chopped dried dates

1. Combine all ingredients in the slow cooker and stir.

2. Cover and cook on low for 6 to 8 hours.

3. This may be a good texture for your weaner, or you can puree in a food processor or blender, adding breast milk or water as needed to achieve the desired consistency.

Slow Cooker Baby Breakfast

1 cup uncooked brown rice, barley, or old-fashioned rolled oats

5 pears, cored, peeled, and diced

4 cups water

1. Combine all ingredients in the slow cooker and stir.

2. Cover and cook on low for 4 to 6 hours.

3. This texture may be perfect for your weaner, or you can puree in a food processor or blender, adding breast milk or water as needed to achieve the desired consistency.

Slow Cooker Meat for Baby

2 pounds boneless, skinless chicken thighs or pork shoulder roast, diced

1 cup water

1. Put the meat and water in the slow cooker.

2. Cover and cook on low for 7 to 9 hours.

3. This texture may be perfect for your weaner, or you can puree in a food processor or blender, adding breast milk or water as needed to achieve the desired consistency.

Slow Cooker Sweet Potatoes and Apples

8–10 apples, peeled, cored, and diced

5 sweet potatoes, peeled and diced

1 cup water

1. Combine all ingredients in the slow cooker and stir.

2. Cover and cook on low for 4 to 6 hours.

3. This texture may be perfect for your weaner, or you can puree in a food processor or blender, adding breast milk or water as needed to achieve the desired consistency.

Slow Cooker Squash, Pears, and Carrots

1 butternut squash, peeled and diced

2 pears, cored and diced

10 carrots, peeled and sliced

½ cup water

1. Combine all ingredients in the slow cooker and stir.

2. Cover and cook on low for 4 to 6 hours.

3. This texture may be perfect for your weaner, or you can puree in a food processor or blender, adding breast milk or water as needed to achieve the desired consistency.

Slow Cooker Pears, Pumpkins, and Apples, Oh My!

3 pears, peeled, cored, and diced

1 pumpkin, cut in half and gutted, flesh scooped out and diced

3 apples, peeled, cored, and diced

1 cup water

1. Combine all ingredients in the slow cooker and stir.

2. Cover and cook on low for 4 to 6 hours.

3. This texture may be perfect for your weaner, or you can puree in a food processor or blender, adding breast milk or water as needed to achieve the desired consistency.

Slow Cooker Apricot Chicken Meal

2 boneless, skinless chicken breasts, diced

10 apricots, peeled, pitted, and chopped

1 cup water

1. Combine all ingredients in the slow cooker and stir.

2. Cover and cook on low for 4 to 6 hours.

3. This texture may be perfect for your weaner, or you can or puree in a food processor or blender, adding breast milk or water as needed to achieve the desired consistency.

Slow Cooker Veggies

1 stalk asparagus, woody end snapped off, chopped

2 sweet potatoes, peeled and cubed

1 butternut squash, peeled, seeded, and cubed

1 red pepper, seeded and cubed

½ cup water

1. Combine all ingredients in the slow cooker and stir.

2. Cover and cook on low for 4 to 6 hours.

3. Cut the veggies into small pieces, or puree in a food processor or blender, adding breast milk or water as needed to achieve the desired consistency.

9–12 Months

💜 Grown-up Grains

💜 Meals & Combos

💜 Finger Foods

🩶 Slow Cooker Recipes

Introduction

It is amazing how quickly you get to this stage! Your weaner will have tried a variety of nutritious foods. They should have the basics of feeding down. This is a great time to start feeding your baby some family meals. This saves you time and your weaner will love eating the same food as an older sibling, mom, or dad! There are a lot of great recipes in this section that the whole family can enjoy.

At 9 months you can also start your baby on dairy! Start with full-fat, plain yogurt, and then try a grated hard cheese. If your weaner tolerates those, and they are eating a variety of foods (including good iron sources), you can introduce full-fat cow's milk between 9 and 12 months.

How Much Can Your Weaner Eat?

This is still not up to you, or us, or your pediatrician. Until 12 months your baby's main source of nutrition is still breast milk and/or formula. As for solids, your weaner will let you know when they are hungry or full at each meal. Feedings will be much more routine than in the beginning, with three regular meals per day. By the time your weaner is 12 months old they can also have 2 or 3 snacks per day.

It is still (and will always be) important to let your weaner choose how much to eat of the foods you offer at each meal. Their appetite is very inconsistent (due to teething, illness, growth spurts, etc.), but it's important to let your weaner grow up listening to their appetite.

Sample Day for a 9-Month-Old

Breakfast	Plain Yogurt + Quinoa, Pears, and Ginger, Oh My! (page 118)
Lunch	Chicken Rice Dish (page 130) + avocado slices
Dinner	Spaghetti and Meatsauce (page 124) + peas

NOTE: Serving sizes have not been given, as this is up to your weaner. Start with a smaller amount, and if they still appear hungry they can have second helpings!

Watch What I Can Do!

At this stage weaners are going to want to start feeding themselves if they haven't already. It is so much fun to watch them manipulate their chunky little fingers and navigate a Toasted O from plate to mouth! They are still getting the hang of using their fine motor skills, so we suggest you still serve your baby from a spoon as well as encourage self-feeding. Or, if they would like to try using the spoon, thicker foods (like oatmeal) will make it easier, as they stick to the spoon. This is also a good time to introduce a small cup at meals with a bit of water, breast milk or fomula.

You can still make your weaner purees but remember it's important to start going a bit chunkier. Just blend less and add less fluid than you did in the earlier stages. You can also keep the peels on some fruits and veggies to add more texture. If you don't introduce some texture into your weaner's diet now, it will be much harder to do it later.

MAMAS BEWARE: This is going to get messy but it's an important step in learning and feeding!

What About Juice?

Juice is not necessary for your weaner. If your weaner is filling up on juice, they may be missing out on some essential nutrients from whole foods, breast milk, or formula. Instead of juice, why not offer a frozen fruit popsicle (page 167) made with whole fruit, as a cool and refreshing treat?

Sugar and Spice: Some of It's Nice!

That's right. You can introduce more spice into your weaner's diet. Added sugar and salt are no-no's the whole way through this book as they are unnecessary for your baby. We don't want them growing up with a sweet or salty tooth if we can help it! If your weaner enjoys more spices than the recipes call for—like cinnamon, nutmeg, oregano and thyme—that's okay, too! Your baby has a more sophisticated palate, so go ahead and add it.

Picky Eaters?

Really, don't stress about this. If your weaner refuses a particular food, try again in a couple of days. If it doesn't work, try again a couple days after that and keep the cycle going. Now is the time to avoid creating a picky eater by introducing as many whole foods as you can. Another important tip to discourage picky eating is to continue letting your weaner choose how much to eat of the foods you offer at each meal. If they are not hungry, there are reasons for that. Your weaner knows his or her own appetite best!

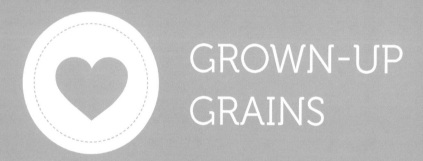

GROWN-UP GRAINS

You can still serve cereal made from powders (pages 19–25), but definitely give these adult-style recipes a try too!

Kamut

1½ cups water

½ cup Kamut

1. Bring the water to a boil in a small saucepan over high heat.

2. Stir in the Kamut, cover the saucepan, and reduce the heat to low.

3. Simmer for 10 minutes.

Quinoa

1½ cups water

½ cup quinoa

1. Bring the water to a boil in a small saucepan over high heat.

2. Stir in the quinoa, cover, and reduce the heat to low.

3. Simmer for 15 minutes, or until the quinoa opens up (like popcorn).

Quinoa, Pears, and Ginger, Oh My!

1¾ cups water

½ cup quinoa

5 pears, cored and diced

1 teaspoon freshly grated ginger

1. Bring the water to a boil in a small saucepan over high heat.

2. Stir in all ingredients, cover, and reduce the heat to low.

3. Simmer for 15 minutes, or until the quinoa opens up (like popcorn).

Blueberry Banana Risotto

1 cup blueberries, cut in half

2 bananas, mashed or cut into small pieces

1 cup Arborio rice, cooked according to package directions

1. Mix all ingredients together.

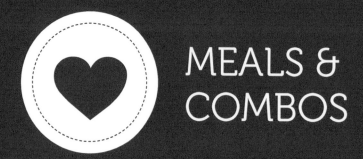

MEALS & COMBOS

The Meals and Combos in the 6–9 month section are still great for your 9–12 month weaner. Just dice or serve whole, instead of pureeing. The following recipes are included in the 9–12 month section because they contain dairy, or have more ingredients. These are great for the baby who loves mixed flavors!

Toasted Eggs

1 slice whole-grain bread

1 teaspoon butter

1 egg yolk or whole egg

1. Using a drinking glass or cookie cutter, cut out a circle from the middle of the bread.

2. In a nonstick skillet, melt the butter over medium-low heat.

3. Place the bread and the cut-out bread circle in the pan.

4. Put the egg yolk (or crack the whole egg) into the hole in the center of the bread.

5. Cover and cook for 5 minutes.

6. Flip both the bread with the egg and the bread circle, and cook for an additional 3 to 5 minutes, or until the egg is set.

7. Top the bread with the cut-out circle.

TIP: This recipe does not make good leftovers!

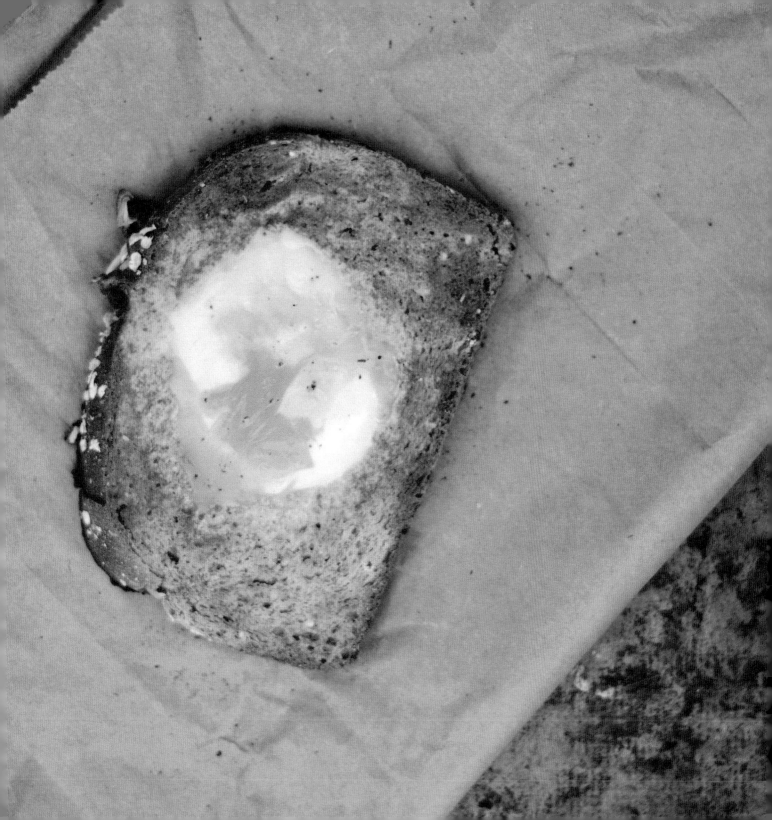

Casserole of Broccoli, Potato, Carrots, and Cheese

Florets from ½ head broccoli, cut into chunks

5 white potatoes, scrubbed and cut into chunks

5 carrots, peeled and cut into chunks

¼ cup grated cheddar cheese

1. Preheat the oven to 400°F.

2. Place the vegetables in a baking dish with just enough water to cover the bottom.

3. Bake for 45 minutes.

4. Add the cheddar cheese and stir until melted.

5. Dice into small pieces if required.

Mashed Potatoes

1 pound white potatoes, peeled and diced

1 tablespoon butter

½ cup cottage cheese

1. Bring a large pot of water to boil over high heat.

2. Add the potatoes and boil for about 20 minutes, or until they break apart easily with a fork.

3. Drain the potatoes in a colander and let cool slightly.

4. Puree the potatoes with the remaining ingredients in a food processor or blender, adding more breast milk or water as needed to achieve the desired consistency.

Scrambled Breakfast

1 egg yolk, or 1 whole egg

1 tablespoon finely chopped red pepper

1 tablespoon finely chopped mushrooms

1 tablespoon grated cheddar cheese

1. Combine the ingredients in a bowl.

2. Pour the mixture into a nonstick or lightly oiled skillet and cook over medium heat until the egg is set, about 5 minutes.

3. Mash the mixture with a fork.

Spaghetti and Meatsauce

½ ripe tomato, diced

¼ onion, diced

1 pound extra-lean ground beef

½ cup homemade bread crumbs
  (see recipe on page 97)

1 cup small-shaped whole-wheat pasta, cooked according to package directions

1. Sauté the tomato and onion in a nonstick or lightly oiled skillet over medium high heat until the onion is translucent, about 5 minutes.

2. Use a slotted spoon to transfer the tomato and onion from the pan to a bowl.

3. Sauté the beef over medium-high heat for 10 minutes, or until cooked through.

4. Stir in the tomato and onion mixture and the breadcrumbs.

5. Pour the meat sauce over the pasta and mix well.

Cucumber Cottage Cheese Snack

½ cucumber, peeled and diced

½ cup cottage cheese

1. Mix the cucumber into the cottage cheese.

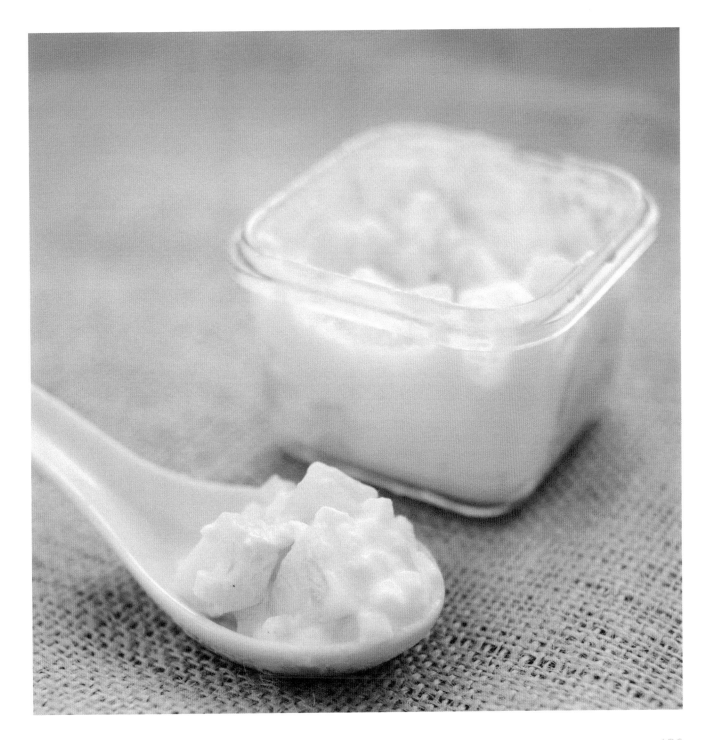

Spinach Salad

1 teaspoon extra-virgin olive oil

1 bunch spinach

1 kiwi, peeled and diced

1 cup blueberries, cut in half

1. Heat the oil in a skillet over medium-high heat.

2. Add the spinach and sauté for 3 to 5 minutes, or until very wilted.

3. Chop the spinach and mix in the kiwi and blueberries.

Sweet Veggies

1 teaspoon extra-virgin olive oil

5 carrots, peeled and chopped

2 celery stalks, chopped

1 cup green beans, ends trimmed

1 teaspoon freshly grated ginger

1 cup raisins

1. Heat the oil in a skillet over medium heat.

2. Add all ingredients and sauté until the veggies are soft, 10 to 15 minutes.

3. Dice into small pieces if required.

Turkey and Carrot Loaf

1 pound lean ground turkey

10 carrots, peeled and grated

1 egg yolk, or 1 whole egg

1. Preheat the oven to 400°F. Lightly grease a loaf pan.

2. Combine all ingredients in a large bowl and mix well.

3. Transfer the mixture to the loaf pan and bake for 50 minutes.

4. Dice into small pieces if required.

Sweet Beefy Veggie Supper

1 cup uncooked lentils

1 teaspoon extra-virgin
olive oil

3 sweet potatoes, peeled
and cut into chunks

5 carrots, peeled and cut
into chunks

1 tomato, chopped

1 cup peas, fresh or frozen

¼ onion, chopped

1 pound extra-lean
ground beef

1. Bring a large pot of water to a boil over high heat.

2. Add the lentils and boil for 30 minutes.

3. Meanwhile, heat the oil in a skillet over medium-high heat.

4. Add the sweet potatoes, carrots, tomato, peas, and onion and sauté for 10 minutes.

5. Push the veggies off to the side of the skillet and add the ground beef. Sauté the beef until brown, about 5 minutes.

6. Stir the veggie mixture into the ground beef and sauté for an additional 10 minutes. Drain lentils, and mix in.

7. Dice into small pieces if required.

Tasty Tofu and Potatoes

1 white potato, scrubbed

4 ounces silken tofu

1 tablespoon water

⅔ cup grated cheddar cheese

1. Preheat the oven to 350°F.

2. Poke the potato seven times with a fork. Place the potato directly on the middle oven rack and bake for 50 minutes.

3. Meanwhile, mash the tofu, water, and cheese together with a fork.

4. Allow the potato to cool slightly. Scoop out the potato from the skin and mash it into the tofu mixture.

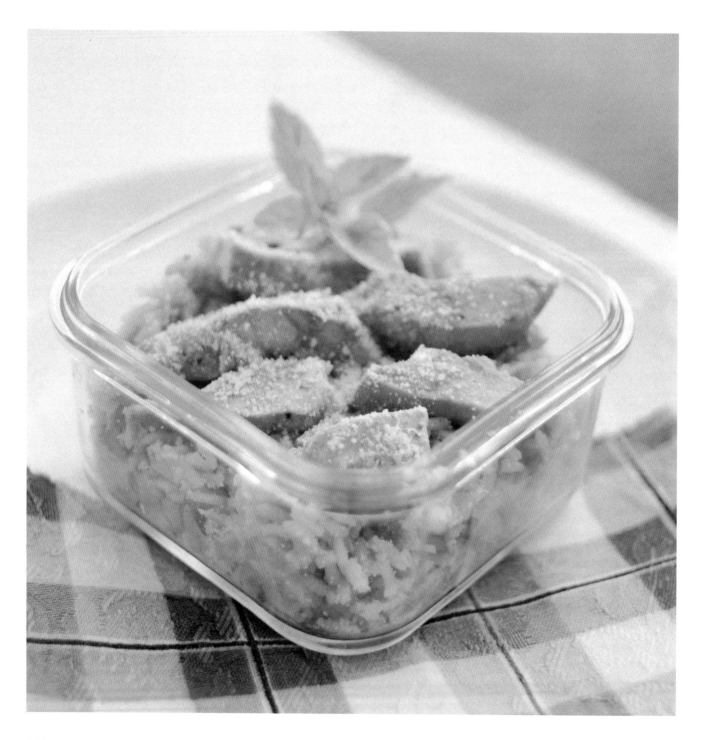

Chicken Rice Dish

1 tablespoon extra-virgin olive oil

½ onion, chopped

2 boneless, skinless chicken breasts, cut into cubes

1 cup uncooked brown rice

2 cups water

1 teaspoon dried basil

1 tablespoon grated Parmesan cheese

1. Heat the oil in a skillet over medium-high heat.

2. Add the onion and sauté for 3 minutes.

3. Add the chicken and cook until brown on all sides, about 3 minutes.

4. Add the rice and 1 cup of the water and stir occasionally until it reduces a bit, about 10 minutes.

5. Add the remaining 1 cup water and continue cooking, stirring occasionally, until the rice is tender, about 25 minutes.

6. Remove from the heat and stir in the basil and Parmesan cheese. Cover and let stand for 5 minutes.

7. Dice into small pieces if required.

Pasta Casserole

2 cups whole-wheat
macaroni, cooked according
to package directions

4 white potatoes, peeled and
cut into chunks

Florets from ½ head broccoli,
chopped

5 carrots, peeled and diced

1 large ripe tomato, diced

1 cup peas, fresh or frozen

Pinch of parsley

1. Preheat the oven to 400°F.

2. Combine the cooked pasta with the rest of the
ingredients in a casserole dish.

3. Cook for 45 to 55 minutes, or until the potatoes are soft.

4. Dice into small pieces if required.

Roast Beef Dinner

1 pound top sirloin roast,
cut into cubes

5 carrots, peeled and cut
into chunks

½ onion, chopped

5 white potatoes, peeled
and cut into chunks

1 cup water

1. Preheat the oven to 325°F.

2. Combine all ingredients in a baking pan.

3. Bake for about 30 minutes, or until your meat
thermometer reads the roast at 160°F.

4. Dice into small pieces if required.

Crustless Chicken Pot Pie

2 cups water

2 boneless, skinless chicken breasts

1 tablespoon butter

1 small onion, diced

2 celery stalks, diced

2 carrots, peeled and diced

½ teaspoon dried thyme

2 tablespoons whole-wheat flour

1 cup breast milk or cow's milk

1 cup peas, fresh or frozen

1. Preheat the oven to 350°F. Lightly grease a 12-cup muffin tin.

2. Place the water and chicken in a medium-size pot and bring the water to a boil over high heat.

3. Reduce the heat to medium-low, partially cover the pot, and simmer for 15 minutes.

4. Transfer the chicken to a plate; reserve the water.

5. Heat ½ tablespoon of the butter in a skillet over medium heat. Add the onion and sauté for 5 minutes, or until translucent.

6. Add the celery, carrots, and thyme and sauté for an additional 5 minutes.

7. Add the remaining ½ tablespoon butter and sprinkle the flour over to make a sauce.

8. Cook for 3 minutes, stirring to coat the vegetables.

9. Add the milk, the reserved chicken cooking water, the chicken, and the peas. Simmer for 10 minutes, or until the mixture is thick and creamy.

10. Divide the mixture into the muffin cups and bake for 30 minutes.

11. Dice into small pieces if required.

Mac 'n' Cheese

*1 cup uncooked whole-wheat
macaroni*

1 large tomato, chopped

¼ cup grated cheddar cheese

1. Bring a medium-size pot of water to a boil over high heat.

2. Add macaroni and tomato.

3. Cook according to package directions (normally around 10 minutes).

4. Drain the water, and stir in the cheese until melted.

5. Dice into small pieces if required.

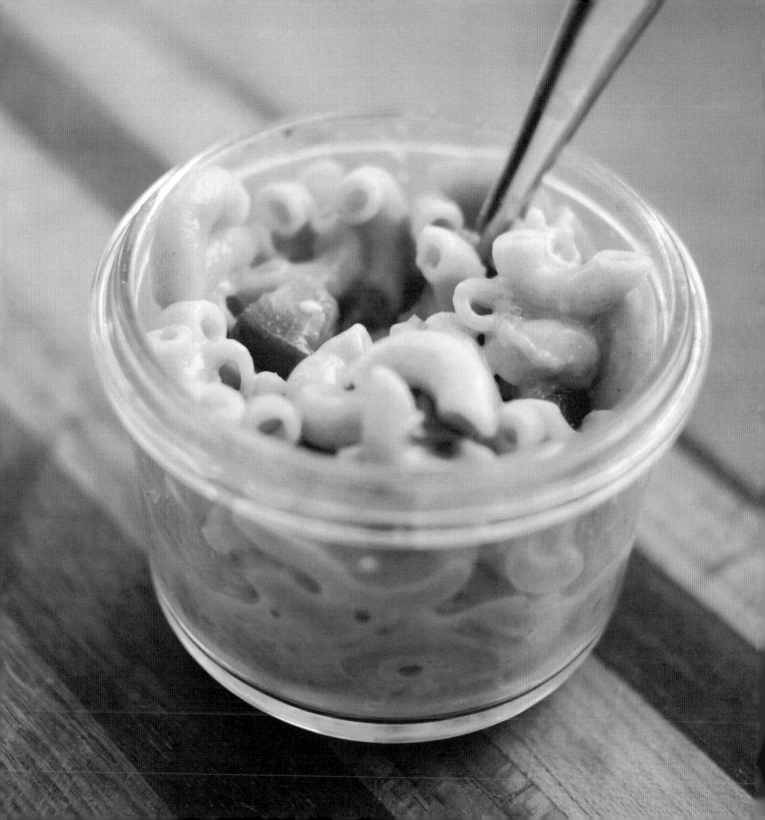

Chicken Meal

2 boneless, skinless chicken breasts, chopped

5 carrots, peeled and chopped

2 sweet potatoes, peeled and chopped

1 pound green beans, ends trimmed, chopped

½ cup water

1. Preheat the oven to 400°F.

2. Combine all ingredients in a casserole dish.

3. Bake for about 30 minutes, or until your meat thermometer reads the chicken at 155°F.

4. Dice into small pieces if required.

Turkey and Veggies

2 boneless, skinless turkey breasts, chopped

5 celery stalks, chopped

1 cup peas, fresh or frozen

3 apples, peeled, cored, and chopped

3 apricots, cut in half and pitted

5 white potatoes, peeled and chopped

1 teaspoon dried parsley

1. Preheat the oven to 400°F.

2. Combine all ingredients in a casserole dish.

3. Cook for 55 minutes, or until your meat thermometer reads 162°F for the turkey.

4. Dice into small pieces if required.

Sweet Chicken

2 boneless, skinless
  chicken breasts

10 apples, peeled, cored,
  and chopped

10 peaches, peeled, pitted,
  and chopped

½ cup water

1. Preheat the oven to 350°F.

2. Place all ingredients in a casserole dish.

3. Bake for about 25 minutes, or until your meat thermometer reads the chicken at 155°F.

4. Dice into small pieces if required.

Pasta Ratatouille

1 cup small whole-grain
  macaroni, cooked according to
  package directions

1 teaspoon extra-virgin olive oil

½ onion, diced

1 eggplant, peeled and diced

1 zucchini, diced

2 large ripe tomatoes, chopped

1 tablespoon chopped fresh basil

¼ cup grated mozzarella cheese

1. Heat the oil in a large skillet over medium heat. Add the onion and sauté for 1 minute.

2. Add the eggplant and zucchini and sauté for 10 minutes. Using a slotted spoon, transfer the veggies to a bowl and set aside.

3. Add the tomatoes to the pan and bring to a boil.

4. Return the veggies to the pan with the tomatoes and add the basil. Reduce the heat to low, and simmer for 5 minutes. Remove from the heat.

5. Add the cooked pasta to the pan and toss to combine with the veggies. Top with the cheese.

6. Dice into small pieces if required.

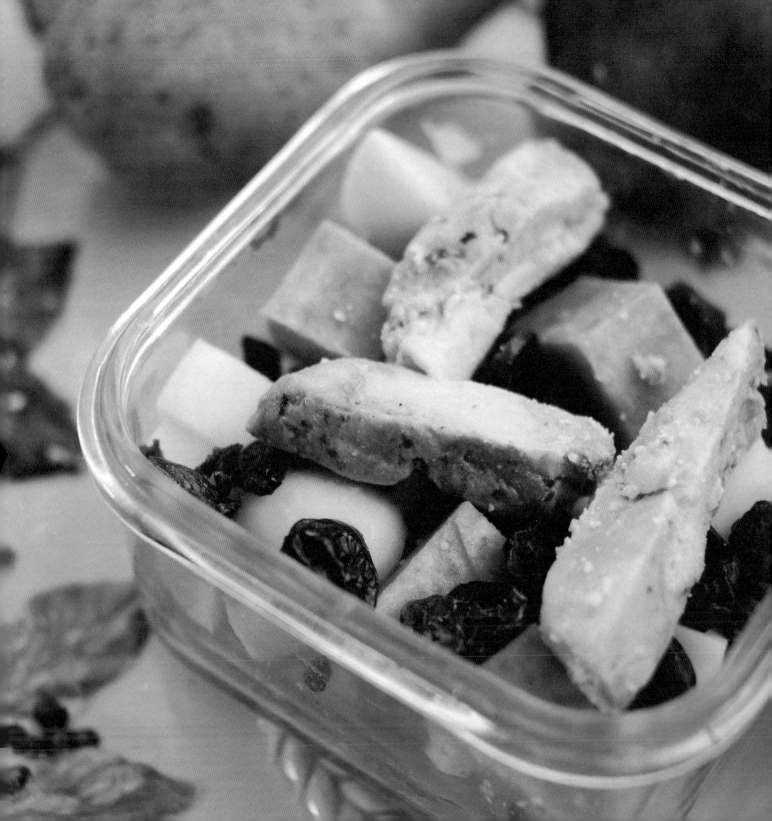

Thankful for
Every Day Feast

2 cups water

2 cups cranberries,
rinsed and picked over

1 sweet potato, peeled
and cubed

2 white potatoes, peeled
and cubed

3 large slices of your
family's cooked turkey

1. Bring the water to a boil in a large pot over high heat.
   Add the cranberries and potatoes.

2. Reduce the heat to low and simmer for 20 minutes. Drain.

3. Add turkey and dice into small pieces if required.

Apple-Turkey Rounds

1 pound ground turkey

2 egg yolks, or 1 whole egg

1 Wean Cube (½ cup) carrot
puree

1 Wean Cube (½ cup) applesauce

1 Wean Cube (½ cup) green bean
puree

¼ cup homemade bread crumbs
(see recipe on page 97)

Pinch of dried basil

1. Preheat the oven to 400°F. Lightly grease a 12-cup muffin tin.

2. Combine all ingredients in a large bowl and mix well.

3. Divide the mixture into the muffin cups and bake for 30 minutes.

4. Dice into small pieces if required.

Scrambled Tofu

8 ounces silken tofu

1 teaspoon extra-virgin olive oil

1 zucchini, diced

¼ cup grated cheddar cheese

1. Squeeze the tofu to remove some of the water.

2. Heat the oil in a skillet over medium-high heat.

3. Add the tofu and zucchini and cook for 10 minutes, mashing as you stir.

4. Top with the cheese.

Crustless Tofu Quiche

1 tablespoon butter, melted

1 cup homemade bread crumbs
(see recipe on page 97)

4 egg yolks or 2 whole eggs

8 ounces silken tofu

1 tablespoon whole-wheat flour

2 teaspoons freshly squeezed
  lemon juice

Pinch of ground nutmeg

Pinch of ground black pepper

¼ cup finely chopped broccoli

¼ cup finely chopped
  cauliflower

¼ cup finely chopped carrots

2 tablespoon grated Parmesan
  cheese

1 medium tomato, cut into
  wedges

1. Preheat the oven to 350°F.

2. Combine the melted butter and bread crumbs in a small bowl. Press the bread crumb mixture onto the bottom of a small pie plate. Set aside.

3. Combine the egg yolks and tofu in a blender or food processor and blend until smooth.

4. Add the flour, lemon juice, nutmeg, and pepper and blend again.

5. Transfer the tofu mixture to a mixing bowl, and stir in the chopped veggies.

6. Pour the tofu mixture into the prepared pie plate and sprinkle with the cheese.

7. Bake for 35 minutes.

8. Arrange the tomato wedges on top and bake for an additional 5 minutes.

9. Dice into small pieces if required.

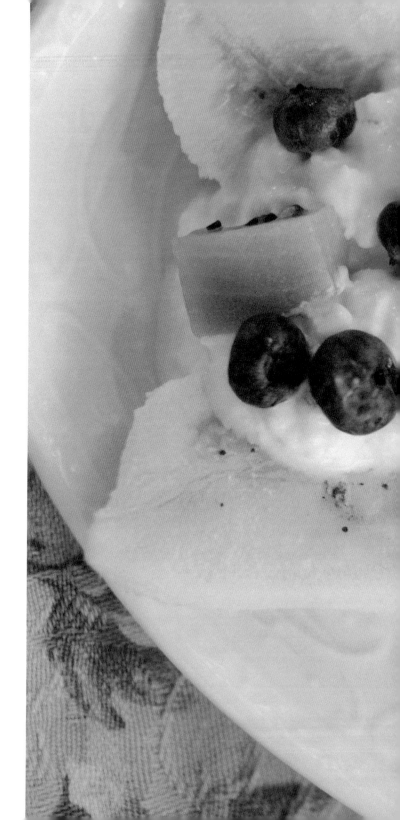

Banana Split

1 banana, peeled and cut in half lengthwise

1 tablespoon cottage cheese

¼ cup blueberries, cut in half

1 kiwi, peeled and chopped

1. Lay the banana halves side by side on a plate.

2. Spread the cottage cheese down the center and pile the fruit on top.

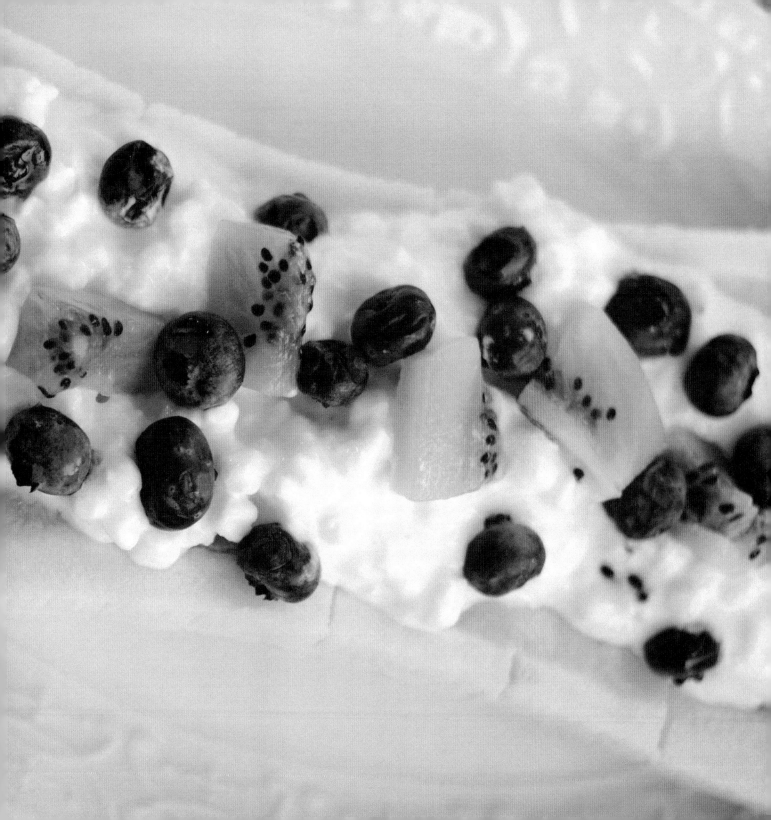

Baby Shepherd's Pie

1 teaspoon extra-virgin olive oil

1 pound extra-lean ground beef

¼ onion, chopped

Pinch of dried parsley

Pinch of dried sage

Pinch of dried thyme

2 cups corn, fresh or frozen

4 or 5 white potatoes, mashed
  (see page 123)

¼ cup grated cheddar cheese

1. Preheat the oven to 375°F.

2. Heat the oil in a large skillet over medium-high heat.

3. Add the ground beef and sauté until browned, about 5 minutes.

4. Add the onion and sauté until soft, about 3 minutes.

5. Stir in the parsley, sage, thyme, and corn.

6. Transfer the beef mixture to a baking dish.

7. Spread the mashed potatoes on top of the beef mixture.

8. Bake for 30 minutes.

9. Sprinkle the cheese on top and bake for an additional 5 minutes.

Baby Stir-Fry

1 teaspoon extra-virgin olive oil

½ onion, diced

Florets from ½ head broccoli, chopped

1 bunch asparagus, woody ends removed, chopped

10 carrots, peeled and chopped

5 mushrooms, scrubbed and chopped

1. Heat the oil in a skillet or wok over medium-high heat.

2. Add the onions, broccoli, asparagus, and carrots and sauté for 5 minutes.

3. Add the mushrooms and sauté for an additional 5 to 10 minutes, or until everything is very soft.

4. Dice into small pieces if required.

Cottage Cheese and Banana

½ cup cottage cheese

1 banana, diced or mashed

1 teaspoon ground cinnamon

1. Mix all ingredients together.

Toasted Os Apple Pie

2 tablespoons butter

1 tablespoon finely
  chopped onion

1 cup Toasted Os cereal,
  coarsely chopped

2 apples, peeled, cored, and
  thinly sliced

5 egg yolks (or 2–3 whole eggs)

1 cup cottage cheese

1 cup grated cheddar cheese

¼ cup water, breast milk,
  or cow's milk

1/8 teaspoon ground nutmeg

1. Preheat the oven to 350°F.

2. In a nonstick skillet, melt the butter over medium heat. Add the onion and sauté for 3 minutes.

3. Remove the skillet from the heat and stir in the Toasted Os cereal.

4. Press the mixture into the bottom and sides of a pie plate to form a crust.

5. Bake for 8 minutes.

6. Meanwhile, bring a large pot of water to a boil over high heat. Add the apples and boil for 4 minutes.

7. Drain the apples well and arrange in the crust.

8. Combine the egg yolks, cottage cheese, cheddar cheese, and milk in a blender or food processor and blend until smooth.

9. Pour the mixture into the crust and sprinkle with the nutmeg.

10. Bake for 45 minutes, or until a toothpick inserted into the center comes out clean.

11. Allow to cool for 10 minutes. Dice into small pieces if required.

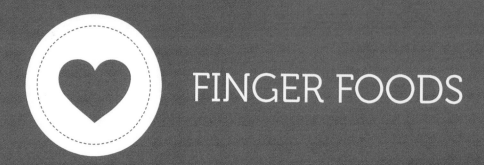

FINGER FOODS

Your weaner's fine motor skills are really developing during this stage. Take advantage of that! While baby serves themselves, you can enjoy a warm meal for the first time in months.

Blueberry Pancakes

1¼ cups breast milk,
  or cow's milk

¾ cup whole-wheat flour

¼ cup wheat germ

2 egg yolks or 1 whole egg, beaten

1 teaspoon baking soda

Pinch of salt

1 cup blueberries

1. Preheat a nonstick or lightly oiled griddle or skillet over medium-high heat.

2. Combine all ingredients in a large bowl and mix well.

3. Pour ¼-cup portions of batter onto the griddle. Flip after 3 to 5 minutes, once they turn golden and begin to bubble. Continue cooking on the second side.

TIP: These freeze great. Thaw them in a toaster oven or microwave.

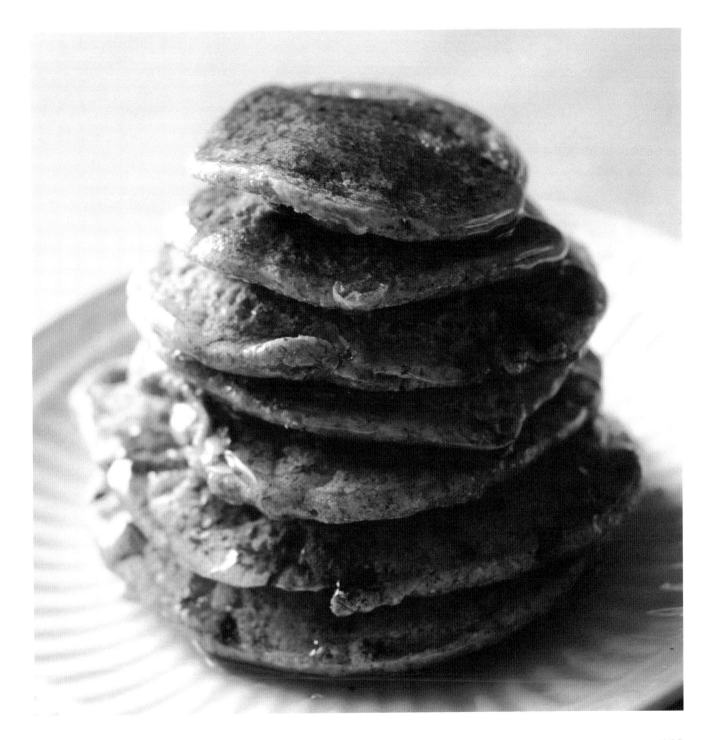

Swiss Tomatoes

1 large, ripe tomato, sliced

Swiss cheese, thinly sliced, 1 piece for each slice of tomato

Pinch of dried or fresh parsley

1. Preheat the oven to 375°F.

2. Place the tomato slices on a nonstick or lightly greased baking sheet.

3. Top each tomato slice with a piece of cheese. Sprinkle with the parsley.

4. Bake for 25 minutes.

5. Dice into small pieces if needed.

Tofu Burgers

8 ounces firm tofu

1 egg or 2 egg yolks

¼ cup homemade bread crumbs
(see recipe on page 97)

¼ onion, diced

1 teaspoon extra-virgin olive oil

1. Combine tofu, egg, bread crumbs, and onion in a blender or food processor and puree.

2. Shape the mixture into about 12 small patties.

3. Heat the oil in a skillet over medium-high heat.

4. Cook the patties for 5 to 8 minutes on each side, or until they are golden brown.

TIP: These are best served warm.

Baked Tofu

8 ounces firm tofu, cubed

5 carrots, peeled and chopped

4 sweet potatoes, peeled and chopped

1. Preheat the oven to 350°F.

2. Combine all ingredients in a baking dish.

3. Bake for 50 minutes, stirring once after 25 minutes.

4. Dice into small pieces if needed.

Wheat Grass Tofu

8 ounces firm tofu, cubed

1 teaspoon minced wheat grass

1. Roll tofu cubes in wheat grass.

Fairy Dust Fruit

1 of your weaner's favorite
fruits, diced

¼ cup wheat germ, wheat bran,
or any cereal powder

1. Roll each piece of fruit in the wheat germ. Now your weaner will get a better grip on that slippery little piece of fruit!

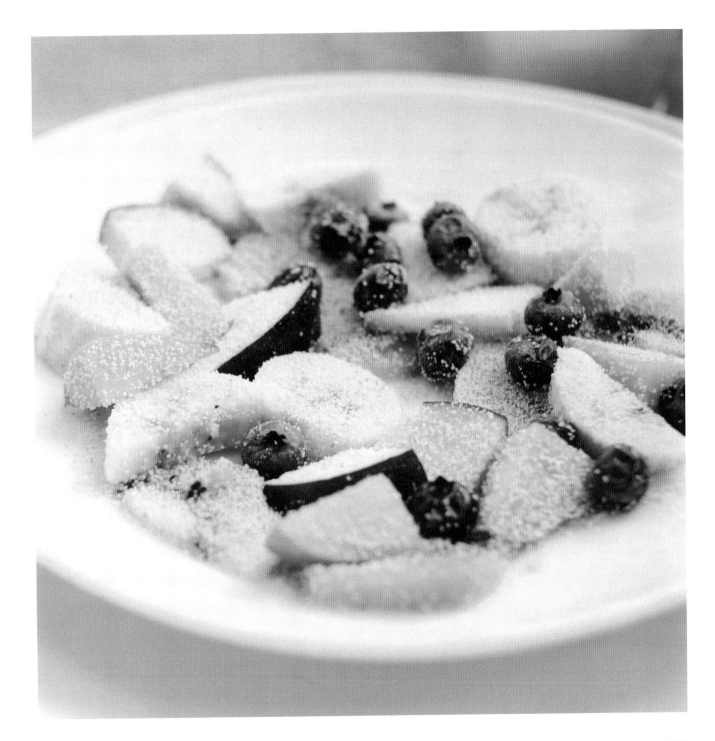

Cinnamony Sweet Potatoes

1 large sweet potato, scrubbed

1 teaspoon ground cinnamon

1. Preheat the oven to 400°F.

2. Poke the sweet potato seven times with a form. Wrap the sweet potato in foil and place directly on the middle oven rack. Bake for 1 hour.

3. Allow to cool slightly. Unwrap the sweet potato, cut in half, and then pull off the skin.

4. Dice the sweet potato and sprinkle with the cinnamon.

Tofu Bites

1 cup finely crushed Toasted Os cereal

1 tablespoon grated Parmesan cheese

Pinch of dried oregano

8 ounces firm tofu, cubed

1 egg yolk, beaten

1. Preheat the oven to 400°F. Lightly grease a baking sheet.

2. Combine the cereal, Parmesan cheese, and oregano on a large plate or sheet of waxed paper.

3. One at a time, dip the tofu pieces in the egg yolk and then roll in the cereal mixture.

4. Place on the prepared baking sheet. Bake for 15 minutes.

TIP: Store leftovers in the fridge for up to 2 days, but do not freeze.

French Toast Fingers

2 egg yolks or 1 whole egg

1 teaspoon ground cinnamon

2 slices whole-grain bread

1 tablespoon canola oil

1. Beat eggs and cinnamon together in a bowl.

2. Coat the bread in the egg mixture.

3. Heat the oil in a large skillet over medium-high heat.

4. Fry bread 3 to 5 minutes on each side, until each side is golden brown.

5. Cut into fingers and serve.

TIP: Store leftovers in the freezer for up to 3 months. Simply pop in your toaster or microwave to thaw them out.

Carrot and Zucchini Patties

3 carrots, peeled and grated

1 zucchini, grated

2 white potatoes, peeled and grated

1 medium onion, grated

2 tablespoons whole-wheat flour

1 egg yolk, beaten

1 teaspoon extra-virgin olive oil

1. Use your hands to squeeze out the excess moisture from the grated veggies.

2. Mix the veggies with the flour and egg and form into small patties, about 3 inches in diameter.

3. Heat the oil in a nonstick skillet over medium-high heat and fry each patty 6 to 8 minutes on each side, or until golden brown.

Sweet Potato Fries

*2 sweet potatoes, peeled and cut
into matchsticks*

1 teaspoon extra-virgin olive oil

1. Preheat the oven to 400°F.

2. Mix the potato sticks with the oil in a
   large boil, tossing to coat.

3. Place the fries on a nonstick baking
   sheet and bake for 40 minutes.

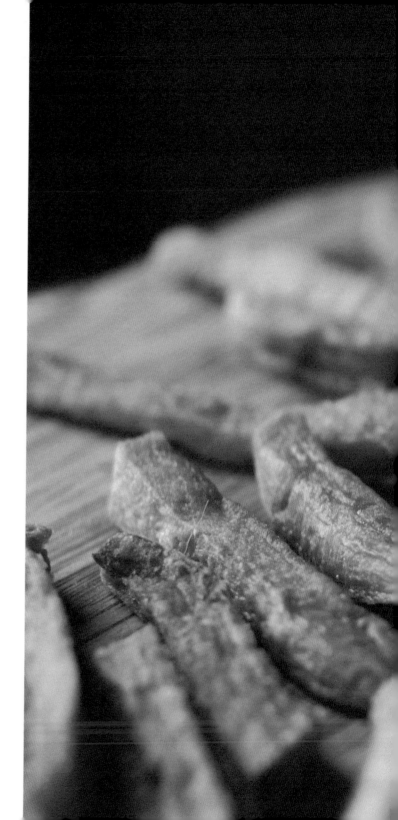

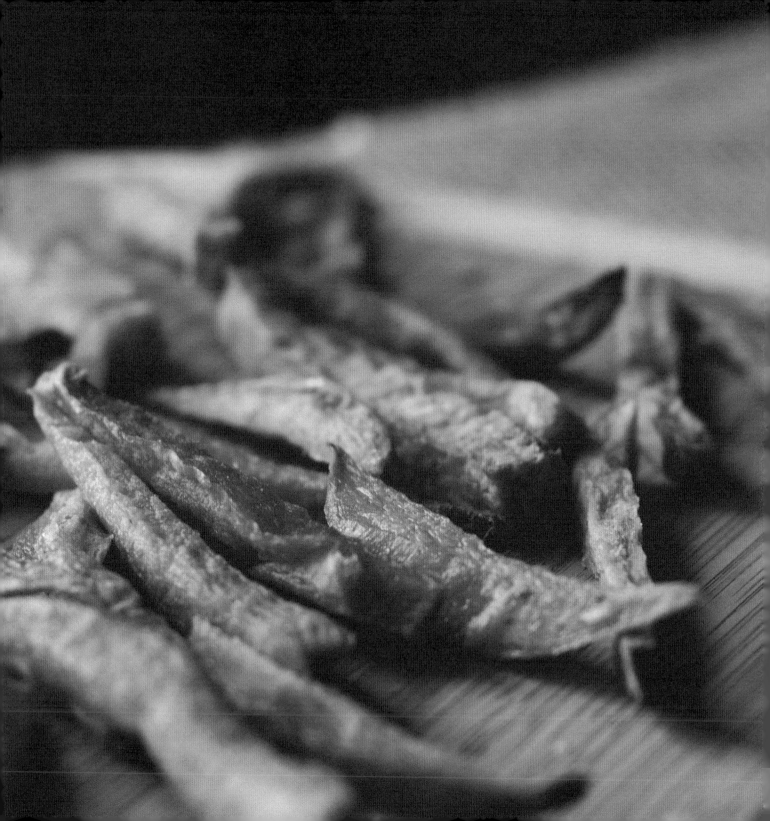

Potato Wedges

4 russet potatoes, scrubbed
and cut into wedges

2 teaspoons extra-virgin
olive oil

1 teaspoon garlic powder

1 teaspoon dried herb blend
(thyme, sage, marjoram)

1. Preheat the oven to 400°F. Line baking sheet(s) with foil.

2. Mix the oil and seasonings in a large bowl. Toss the potatoes with the oil mixture.

3. Place the potatoes on the prepared baking sheet.

4. Bake for 20 minutes, and then flip the potatoes.

5. Bake for an additional 20 minutes, or until the potatoes are crisp on the outside and tender on the inside.

Chapatti (Tasty Indian Bread)

1½ cups whole-wheat flour

¾ cup all-purpose flour

Pinch of salt

1 cup water

1 teaspoon vegetable oil

1. Combine the flours and salt in a large mixing bowl.

2. Add the water a little at a time, mixing the dough with a spoon, until it starts to form into a ball.

3. Knead the dough for 5 minutes. Place a clean, damp towel over the dough and let it rest for 30 minutes.

4. Divide the dough into 12 pieces. Knead each piece into a flat circle.

5. In a large skillet, heat oil over medium-high heat.

6. Add the chapatti dough to the skillet. Cook until the bread puffs up slightly and starts to brown, about 5 minutes. Flip them over, and then cook the other side. Add more oil to pan if extra batches are required, and pan is dry.

Chicken Fingers

1 boneless, skinless chicken breast, cut into strips

4 tablespoons plain yogurt

½ cup homemade bread crumbs
(see recipe on page 97)

1 teaspoon grated Parmesan cheese

Pinch of dried basil

Pinch of dried thyme

1. Preheat the oven to 400°F. Lightly grease a baking dish.

2. In a medium-size bowl, roll the chicken strips in the yogurt until coated.

3. Combine the remaining ingredients in another bowl. Toss the yogurt-covered chicken in the bread crumb mixture until coated on all sides.

4. Place the chicken on the prepared baking dish and bake for 15 minutes, turning the chicken over after 8 minutes. The fingers are done when the breading is toasted brown, and your meat thermometer reads the chicken at 155°F.

5. Dice into small pieces if required.

TIP: Are you looking for a dipping sauce? The Roasted Apple Puree (page 49) tastes great with chicken!

Graham Crackers

2½ cups graham flour

1 cup whole-wheat flour

1 teaspoon salt

½ teaspoon baking powder

1 teaspoon ground cinnamon

¼ cup (½ stick) butter

½ cup lightly packed brown sugar

1 teaspoon pure vanilla extract

⅓ cup full-fat cow's milk

⅓ cup water

1. Mix the flours, salt, baking powder, and cinnamon in a medium-size bowl.

2. In a separate bowl, use an electric mixer to beat the butter and sugar until fluffy.

3. Mix the vanilla into the butter-sugar mixture.

4. Combine the milk and water in a cup.

5. Add half of the flour mixture to the butter mixture and blend well.

6. Add half of the milk-water mixture to the bowl and continue to blend well.

7. Add the rest of the flour mixture, still blending.

8. Add the rest of the milk-water mixture to the bowl and blend. If dough is too dry and crumbly, continue to add water, 1 tablespoon at a time, until it forms a dough ball.

9. Turn off the mixer and let the dough sit at room temperature for 30 minutes. Preheat the oven to 350°F. Lightly grease a cookie sheet.

10. On a floured surface, roll the dough out to ½ inch thick.

11. Place the dough on a prepared cookie sheet.

12. Using a pizza wheel or sharp knife, cut the dough into squares. No need to separate them now, as you will break them apart after cooking.

13. Bake for 30 minutes, or until the squares are browned. Cool in the pan, and break apart into crackers.

TIP: Store graham crackers in an airtight container at room temperature for up to 1 month.

Broccoli Bites

2 cups broccoli florets

1 cup homemade bread crumbs
(see recipe on page 97)

1 cup grated cheddar cheese

4 egg yolks, or 2 whole eggs

Pinch of dried basil

Pinch of dried oregano

1. Preheat the oven to 350°F. Lightly grease a baking sheet.

2. Place a steamer basket in a pot and add enough water to just touch the bottom of the steamer basket.

3. Cover the pot and bring the water to a boil over high heat.

4. Add the broccoli, turn the heat down to medium, and loosely cover the pot.

5. Steam for 3 to 5 minutes, or until the broccoli is very soft.

6. Combine the cooked broccoli, bread crumbs, cheese, egg yolks, basil, and oregano in a large bowl, stirring well.

7. Drop teaspoon-size portions of the mixture onto the prepared baking sheet.

8. Bake for 10 minutes, flip them over, and bake an additional 10 minutes.

9. Dice into small pieces if required.

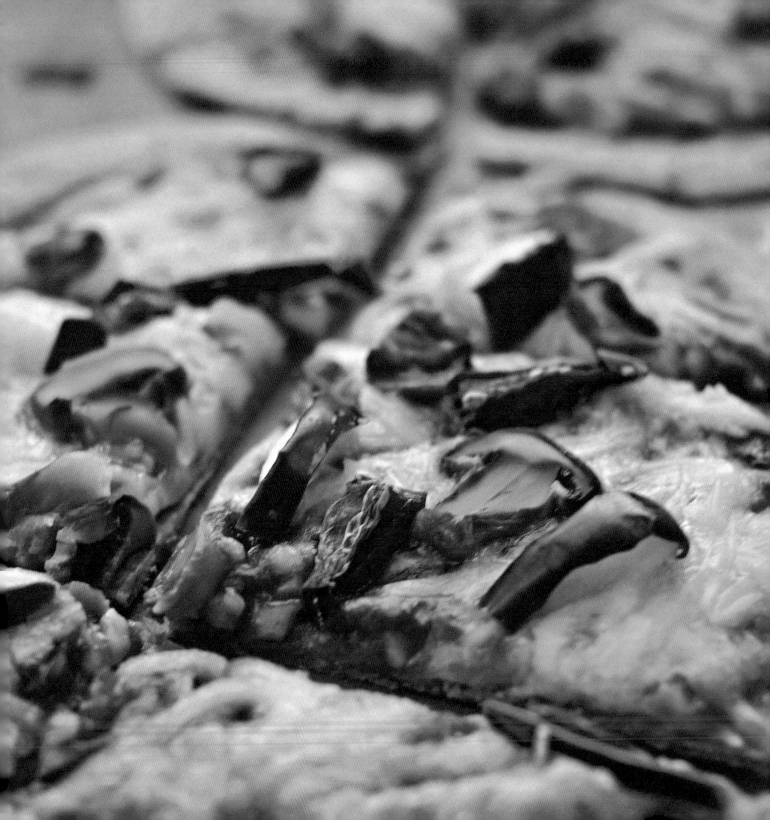

Baby Veggie Pizza

¼ cup marinara sauce

2 whole-wheat tortillas

¼ red bell pepper, diced

¼ zucchini, diced

3 mushrooms,
  scrubbed and diced

½ cup grated mozzarella cheese

Pinch of dried basil

1. Preheat the oven to 375°F.

2. Spread the marinara sauce on the tortillas.

3. Top with the peppers, zucchini, mushrooms, and then the cheese. Sprinkle with the basil.

4. Place on a baking sheet and bake for 8 minutes. Remove the pizzas from the oven and turn the oven up to broil.

5. Broil for 2 minutes.

6. Dice into small pieces if required.

Meatballs

1 cup **Mashed Potatoes**
(see recipe on page 123)

1 pound **extra-lean ground beef
or bison**

1 teaspoon **dried parsley**

1. Preheat the oven to 375°F.

2. Combine the mashed potatoes, beef, and parsley in a large bowl and mix well.

3. Roll the beef mixture into balls and place in a nonstick or lightly greased baking pan.

4. Bake for 25 minutes.

5. Dice into small pieces if required.

Egg Wrap

1 **egg yolk or whole egg**

¼ cup **grated cheddar cheese**

½ **Wean Cube (¼ cup)
broccoli puree**

1 **whole-wheat tortilla**

1. Heat a small nonstick or lightly oiled skillet over medium-high heat. Add the egg and cook, stirring until set, 2 to 3 minutes.

2. Combine the egg, cheese, and broccoli in a small bowl and mix well.

3. Spread the mixture on the tortilla and roll it up.

Shish Kebobs

3 cherry tomatoes

3 cubes cheddar cheese

*½ green pepper,
cut into 3 chunks*

*1 slice whole-grain bread,
toasted and cut into 9 squares*

1. Preheat the broiler. Line a baking sheet with foil.

2. On two metal or soaked wooden skewers, alternate tomatoes, cheese, peppers, and toast squares.

3. Place the skewers on the prepared baking sheet and broil for 3 minutes per side.

4. Bake for 10 minutes, flip them over, and bake an additional 10 minutes.

5. Dice into small pieces if required.

Veggie and Cheese Grilled Sandwich

*½ Wean Cube (¼ cup)
broccoli puree, thawed*

*½ Wean Cube (¼ cup) carrot
puree, thawed*

1 teaspoon butter

2 slices whole-grain bread

2 to 3 slices cheddar cheese

1. Mix together the thawed broccoli and carrot purees.

2. Spread the pureed veggies on one slice of bread. Place the cheese on top, and close it up with the other slice of bread.

3. Butter the outside of each slice of bread.

4. Heat a small skillet over medium-high heat.

5. Cook the sandwich for 2 minutes on each side.

Snack Mix

1 teaspoon butter

1½ cups Toasted Os cereal

½ cup broken
  low-sodium pretzels

½ cup finely chopped raisins

1. In a large nonstick skillet, melt the butter over medium-low heat.

2. Add the cereal and cook, stirring constantly, for 5 minutes.

3. Remove from the heat and let cool.

4. Stir in the pretzels and raisins.

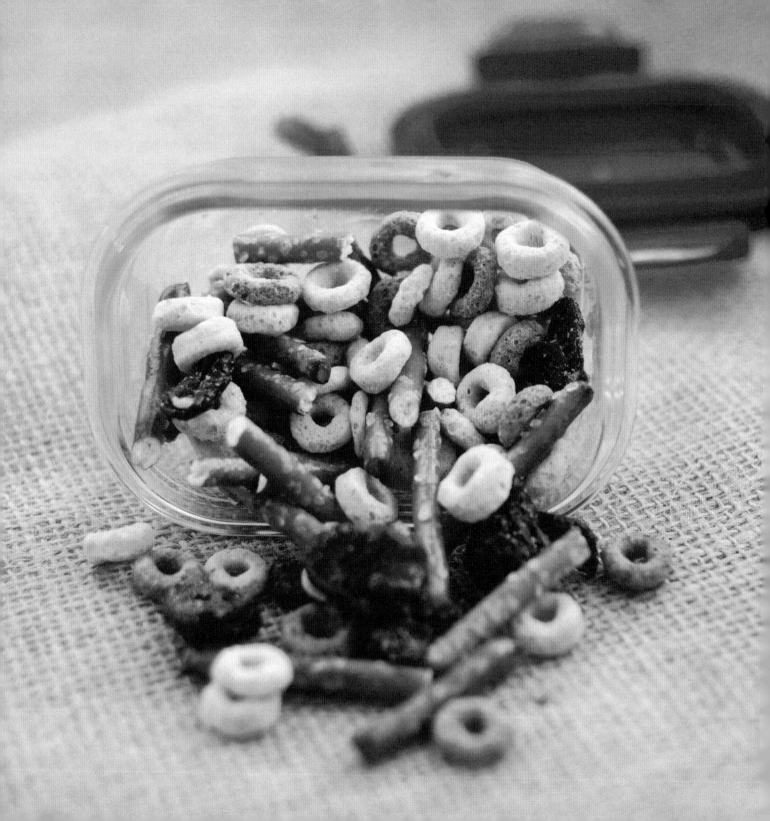

Fruit Popsicles

1 cup cherries, pitted

2 ripe pears, peeled, cored, and cut into chunks

1. Blend the cherries and pears together in a blender or food processor.

2. Fill each Wean Cube.

3. Put a popsicle stick in the center of each cube.

4. Freeze overnight before serving.

TIP: These popsicles can be stored in the freezer for up to 4 months.

Chicken and Apple Rolls

2 boneless, skinless chicken breasts

1 large apple, peeled, cored, and grated

½ small onion, chopped

1 teaspoon dried sage

1 low-sodium chicken bouillon cube, crushed

2 tablespoons homemade bread crumbs

(see recipe on page 97)

1. Preheat the oven to 375°F. Line a cookie sheet with foil.

2. Chop the chicken very finely in your food processor.

3. Combine the chicken, apple, onion, sage, bouillon, and bread crumbs in a large bowl.

4. Using an ice cream scoop, scoop balls of the mixture onto the prepared cookie sheet.

5. Bake for 20 minutes.

6. Dice into small pieces if required.

TIP: This is a great recipe for the whole family. If the balls are too dry for big kids and parents, you can serve them with spaghetti and marinara sauce.

Veggie Dip

½ cup plain yogurt

¼ cucumber, peeled
   and minced

1 teaspoon dried dill
   or 1 tablespoon chopped
   fresh dill

1 teaspoon garlic powder

1. Combine all ingredients and chill for one hour.

TIP: This dip tastes great with cucumber sticks and cauliflower!

Chicken Quesadillas

1 boneless, skinless
   chicken breast

1 teaspoon extra-virgin olive oil

½ yellow pepper, diced

¼ onion, diced

1 ripe tomato, diced

½ cup grated mozzarella cheese

2 whole-wheat tortillas

1. Preheat the oven to 350°F.

2. Place the chicken in a baking dish and bake for 25 minutes or until your meat thermometer reads the chicken at 155°F.

3. Meanwhile, in a nonstick skillet, heat the oil over medium-high heat and sauté the pepper and onion until soft, about 5 minutes.

4. Shred the cooked chicken with your fingers or two forks. Combine the chicken, pepper, onion, tomato, and cheese in a large bowl.

5. Lay 1 tortilla flat in a skillet.

6. Spread the chicken mixture on half of each tortilla and fold in half.

7. Turn the heat to medium and fry the quesadillas until each side is slightly crisp, about 5 minutes per side.

8. Dice into small pieces if required.

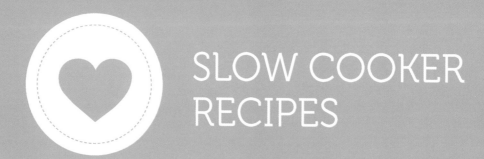

SLOW COOKER
RECIPES

Slow Cooker Peachy Carrots

5 peaches, pitted and diced

10 carrots, peeled and diced

1 cup water

1. Combine all ingredients in the slow cooker and stir.

2. Cook on low for 4 to 6 hours.

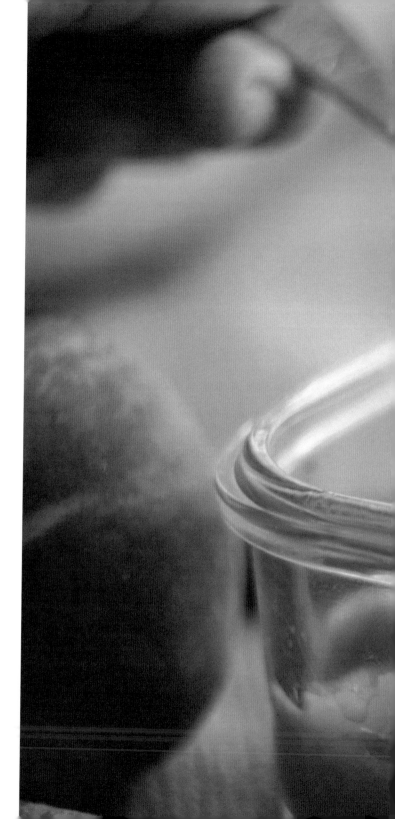

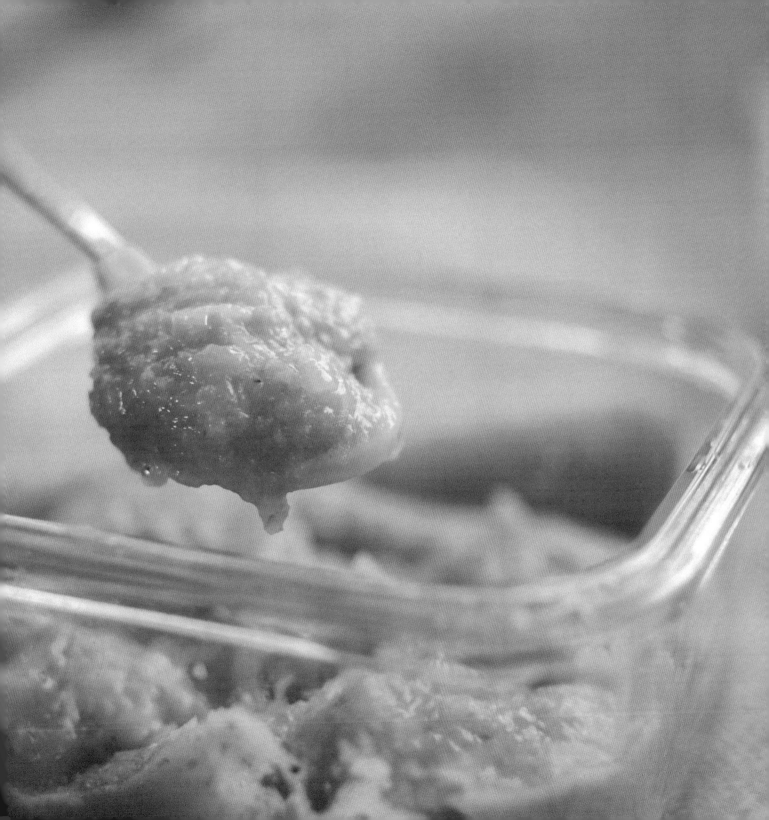

Slow Cooker Apple Delight Breakfast

1 cup breast milk, or cow's milk

1 cup water

Pinch of brown sugar

1 teaspoon butter

Pinch of salt

1 teaspoon ground cinnamon

1 cup old-fashioned rolled oats

3 apples, peeled, cored, and diced

½ cup chopped dried dates

1. Combine all ingredients in the slow cooker and stir.

2. Cover and cook on low for 4 to 6 hours.

Slow Cooker Roast Beef Dinner

1 pound top sirloin roast

5 carrots, peeled and chopped

1 onion, chopped

2 white potatoes,
    peeled and chopped

1 teaspoon garlic powder

1 teaspoon onion powder

1 cup water

1. Place the roast in the slow cooker.

2. Put the veggies on top of the roast.

3. Sprinkle the garlic and onion powders over all.

4. Pour in the water.

5. Cover and cook on low for 6 to 8 hours.

Slow Cooker Chicken and Rice Supper

1 cup short-grain brown rice

2 boneless, skinless chicken
    breasts, diced

3 large carrots,
    peeled and diced

½ cup peas, fresh or frozen

6 cups water

1. Combine all ingredients in the slow cooker and stir.

2. Cover and cook on low for 7 to 9 hours.

3. Drain any extra water, if required.

Slow Cooker Eggplant Quinoa

1 cup quinoa

1 large eggplant, peeled and diced

2½ cups water

1. Combine all ingredients in the slow cooker and stir.

2. Cover and cook on low for 6 to 8 hours.

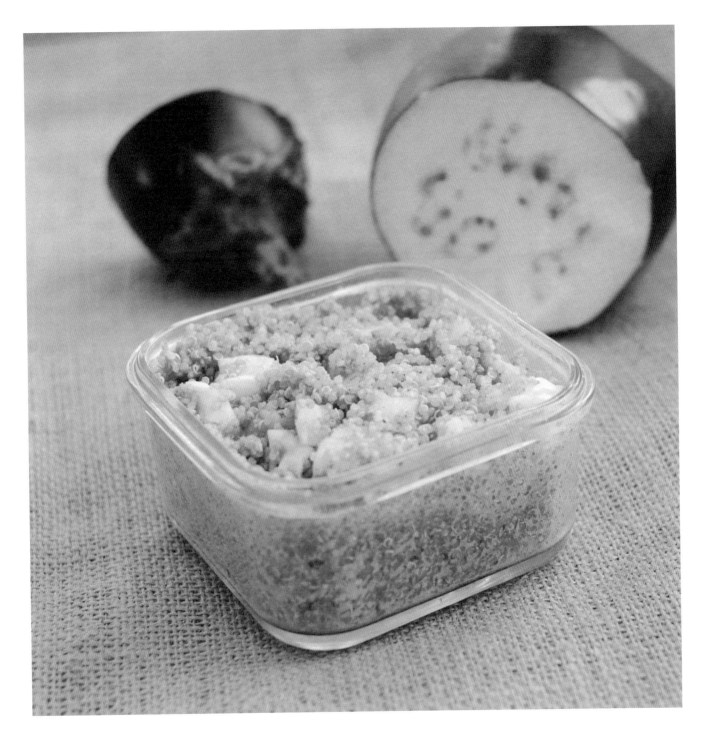

Slow Cooker Acorn Squash and Persimmons

1 large acorn squash, cut in half and seeded, flesh scooped out and diced

5 persimmons, peeled and diced

1 cup water

1. Combine all ingredients in the slow cooker and stir.

2. Cover and cook on low for 4 to 6 hours.

Slow Cooker Plummed Chicken

5 plums, peeled, pitted, and diced

2 boneless, skinless chicken breasts, diced

1 cup water

1. Combine all ingredients in the slow cooker and stir.

2. Cover and cook on low for 7 to 9 hours.

Slow Cooker
Parsnip Mix Lunch

1 pound parsnips, peeled
   and chopped

5 apples, peeled, cored,
   and chopped

1 cup brown rice

1 teaspoon wheat germ

2 cups water

1. Combine all ingredients in the slow cooker and stir.

2. Cover and cook on low for 6 to 8 hours.

Slow Cooker Baby Stew

1 boneless, skinless chicken
   breast or 1 pound lean
   stew beef, diced

5 carrots, peeled and diced

½ onion, diced

3 white potatoes, peeled
   and diced

1 cup peas, fresh or frozen

4 cups water

1. Combine all ingredients in the slow cooker and stir.

2. Cover and cook on low for 7 to 9 hours.

3. Drain any extra water, if required.

Index

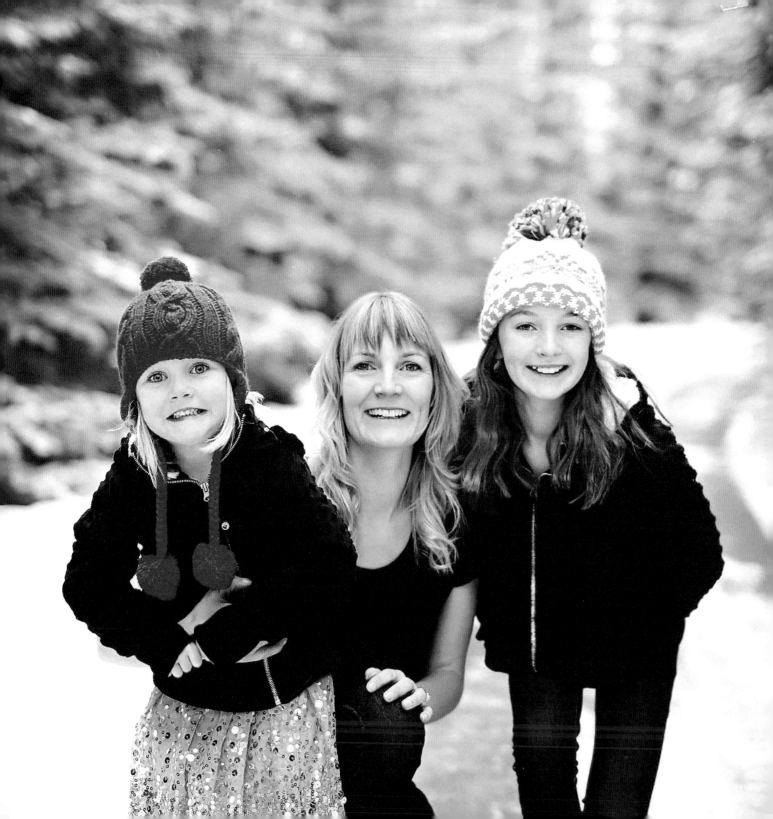

About the Author

Wean Green was founded in 2008 by Melissa Gunning, the proud mom of two little weaners, Rayne and Talia. Melissa's passion for healthy living and happy babies was channeled into Wean Green; creating a company dedicated to providing parents with safe and environmentally friendly products.

Understanding that convenience and 'cool factor' play a role in making the entire family happy, Wean Green has great style and fits easily into diaper bags, on-the-go bags, and backpacks!

Wean Green is devoted to combining eco and chic in all of their products. The eco-chic designs make it possible for parents to choose sustainable products without sacrificing style.

Wean Green's goal is to ensure your eco-footprint does not grow faster than your baby's sweet little feet. The Wean Green team continues to design products that meet the expectations of little weaners, bigger kids and their proud parents.

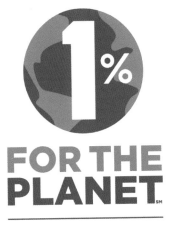

MEMBER

Giving back to the environment

Wean Green is proud to partner with 1% For the Planet, an organization dedicated to building and supporting an alliance of businesses financially committed to creating a healthy planet.

For more information on the work we support, visit **onepercentfortheplanet.org**

Made in the USA
Charleston, SC
17 February 2014